Anesthesiology Simulation

Claire Sampankanpanich Soria • Phil Yao

Editors

Anesthesiology Simulation

A Complete Education Guide for Instructors and Trainees

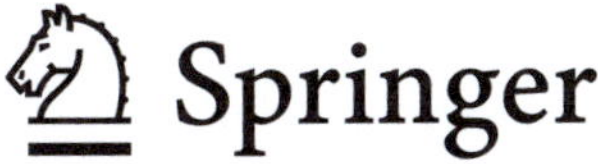

Editors
Claire Sampankanpanich Soria
University of California, San Diego
San Diego, CA, USA

Phil Yao
Pediatric Anesthesiology
Seattle Children's Hospital
Seattle, WA, USA

ISBN 978-3-031-80230-0   ISBN 978-3-031-80228-7   (eBook)
https://doi.org/10.1007/978-3-031-80228-7

This Springer imprint is published by the registered company Springer Nature Switzerland AG
The registered company address is: Gewerbestrasse 11, 6330 Cham, Switzerland

If disposing of this product, please recycle the paper.

Contents

Trauma Burn Airway

1

Caitlin Krol and Claire Sampankanpanich Soria

1.1 Level of Training

- Anesthesiology resident
- General surgery resident

1.2 Learning Objectives

1. Discuss how to recognize and manage extensive thermal burns with airway involvement, including the potential for surgical airway management.
2. Review how to address initial fluid management in the burn patient.
3. Identify potential toxic exposures in a burn patient.

1.3 Simulator Environment

1. Location: trauma bay of an adult hospital.
2. Manikin setup:
    (a) Age: adult.
    (b) Lines: 1 × 18 G peripheral intravenous line (PIV) in antecubital fossa (AC).
    (c) Monitors: non-invasive blood pressure (NIBP) cuff, 5-lead electrocardiogram (EKG), pulse oximeter.
3. Medications available:
    (a) Fluids: normal saline, lactated ringers, albumin.
    (b) Sedatives/hypnotics: propofol, etomidate, ketamine, inhaled anesthetics.
    (c) Paralytics: succinylcholine, rocuronium.

C. Krol (✉) · C. S. Soria
University of California, San Diego, San Diego, CA, USA
e-mail: ckrol@health.ucsd.edu; cssoria@health.ucsd.edu

© The Author(s), under exclusive license to Springer Nature Switzerland AG 2024
C. S. Soria, P. Yao (eds.), *Anesthesiology Simulation*,
https://doi.org/10.1007/978-3-031-80228-7_1

    (d) Cardiac agents: epinephrine, phenylephrine, ephedrine, vasopressin, atropine, glycopyrrolate, esmolol, labetalol, nicardipine, dopamine.

    (e) Narcotics: midazolam, fentanyl, hydromorphone.

4. Equipment available:

    (a) Airway equipment: Mapleson circuit, Ambu bag, laryngoscope, and cuffed ETTs of various sizes, stylet, oral airway, nasal trumpet, laryngeal mask airway (LMA), bougie. GlideScope and fiber optic tower are available if asked for.

    (b) Monitors: pulse oximeter, blood pressure (BP) cuff, 5-lead EKG, end-tidal carbon dioxide ($ETCO_2$) monitor.

    (c) Lines: arterial line kit and transducer, central line kit, and PIV kits are available upon request.

    (d) Crash cart with a defibrillator in the trauma bay is available upon request.

1.4 Actors

1. Emergency medical services/firefighter team
2. Trauma nurses
3. Respiratory therapists
4. Emergency medicine physician
5. Trauma surgeon
6. Anesthesiologist

1.5 Case Narrative

1. Background:

    (a) You are the anesthesiologist team and surgical team on call. You are both called STAT to the trauma bay for a house fire.

2. Case scenario (information provided upfront to the learners):

    (a) Upon arrival, you see a 50-year-old male brought in by firefighters/ emergency medical services (EMS) team. The room smells of smoke.

    (b) The EMS team gave a report: there was a large fire noted by an upstairs tenant. They attempted to enter the apartment but were unsuccessful. EMS was called. Fire rescue arrived first and found the patient passed out on the floor of his apartment. He was covered in vomit with bottles of alcohol noted to be around him as well as lit cigarettes/joints, which appeared to have started the fire. Cardiopulmonary resuscitation (CPR)was required for 2 min. Return of spontaneous circulation (ROSC) was achieved. One dose of naloxone was administered in the field.

    (c) In the trauma bay, the patient is drowsy but has regained a pulse, a BP, and is initiating spontaneous respiratory effort.

3. Additional case information (information to be provided only as specifically requested by learners during initial trauma survey, focused history/physical examination):
   (a) The patient is unable to provide any information. Allergies, medications, past medical history, and past surgical history are unknown.
   (b) Current vital signs: heart rate (HR) 130 bpm, BP 90/60 mmHg, oxygen saturation (SpO_2) 93% on 100% FiO_2 non-rebreather, temperature (T) 37.8 °C, respiratory rate (RR) 26 bpm and shallow.
   (c) Physical exam: measured height and weight unable to be done in the trauma bay, but appears to be 6′, 100 kg, body mass index (BMI) 30. C-collar in place. He is covered in soot. There is vomit around his mouth, soot inside and outside of his nose and mouth, and his eyebrows are singed. The face appears red and swollen.
   (d) Trauma survey: estimated 60% total body surface area (TBSA) second- and third-degree burns. Neurologic exam: extraocular movements intact, though the patient is not very cooperative, pupils pinpoint, Glasgow coma scale (GCS) score of 8. Cardiovascular: tachycardic, regular rhythm, no murmurs. Respiratory: spontaneous shallow breathing, bilateral end-expiratory wheezing on auscultation. Abdomen: soft with abdominal wall burns. Extremities: burns on anterior and posterior extremities.

1.6 Scenario Development

1. Phase 1: Initial survey and resuscitation
   (a) The learners should identify a team leader and delegate tasks efficiently and effectively. Typically, the trauma surgeon is the team leader in the trauma bay. If and when the anesthesiologist determines the patient needs to be intubated, the anesthesiologist and surgeon need to discuss when, where, and how this should be done, including consideration of anticipated difficult airway, hemodynamic instability, and other traumatic injuries that need to be treated.
   (b) The team leader should perform a rapid ABCDE assessment and brief history (consider AMPLE).
       • ABCDE: Airway, Breathing, Circulation, Disability, Exposure.
       • AMPLE: Allergies, Medications, Past medical history, Last oral intake, Events leading to Present Illness or Injury.
   (c) The team should check that monitors are on the patient, including a 5-lead EKG, NIBP cuff, oxygen saturation (SpO_2), and skin thermometer.
   (d) The respiratory therapist should work with the anesthesiologist at the head of the bed to administer supplemental oxygen, perform an airway exam, and prepare for advanced airway, namely a timely intubation.
   (e) The team should obtain additional intravascular (IV) access such as large-bore peripheral IVs or central lines. Additional monitoring and access for such an extensive burn should also be an arterial line, which may be done

    peripherally such as in a radial or dorsalis pedis artery or in a larger artery such as the femoral artery.

(f) The team should perform IV fluid resuscitation. This may be done empirically as a fluid bolus of crystalloid 20–40 cc/kg to start, with repeated boluses as needed to treat tachycardiac and hypotension. The team may also calculate fluid bolus volume based on the Parkland formula: a total of 4 cc/kg/TBSA × % TBSA burned × patient body weight (kg), with half administered in the first 8 h and the second half administered in the next 16 h. This is also titrated to hypotension, tachycardia, and urine output, with a goal urine output >0.5 cc/kg/h.

(g) While obtaining vascular access, the team should draw a rainbow panel of labs, including complete blood count (CBC), complete metabolic panel (CMP), arterial blood gas (ABG), lactate, coagulation panel, type and screen/type and cross, blood cultures, urine cultures, urinalysis, troponin level, and urine toxicology screen. The team may also consider carboxyhemoglobin levels.

(h) While managing the airway and repositioning the patient for examination or procedures, the team should be cognizant of cervical spine precautions.

(i) The team leader should calculate the percent TBSA of the burns, including their depth and location. This will impact fluid resuscitation, anticipated transfusion requirements, and potential need for urgent versus emergent intubation, fasciotomy, and/or escharotomy.

(j) The team should perform imaging studies in the trauma bay, including chest X-ray, and consider a focused assessment of sonography in trauma (FAST) exam. The team may consider additional imaging studies including a computed tomography (CT) scan of the head, but may defer this until later pending examination and hemodynamic instability.

2. Phase 2: Airway management

(a) Identify the patient's risk of having or developing airway edema and lung injury due to smoke inhalation.

(b) The team should also consider aspiration risk given recent substance abuse and poor mental status exam.

(c) The team should recognize that this patient has sustained smoke inhalation injury (evidence: soot in the nose and mouth, wheezing on auscultation, erythematous swollen face) and is likely to decompensate quickly. He is at high aspiration risk and high risk of becoming difficult if not impossible to bag mask ventilate or intubate if intubation is delayed. This will likely be initiated by the anesthesia team but should be communicated in a timely fashion to the trauma surgery team running the trauma resuscitation.

(d) In joint decision-making with the trauma surgeons, the anesthesiologists should proceed with timely intubation. As a team, they may decide to quickly establish large-bore IV access, arterial line placement, and fluid resuscitation as quickly as possible prior to induction and intubation. This will decrease the risk of profound hemodynamic instability following sympathectomy from induction medications. However, if the team decides the patient is devolving into respiratory failure too quickly, they may choose to intubate sooner.

(e) The anesthesiologist should ensure appropriate airway supplies are available including difficult airway equipment. The learner must clearly communicate what staff and equipment they need; otherwise, it will not be provided in the scenario.

- Mnemonics used for airway setup include MOMSAID: Machine (Mapleson, Ambu bag), Oxygen, Monitors, Suction, Airway, IV, and Drugs.
- Standard airway equipment will include various sizes and types of straight and curved laryngoscopes for direct laryngoscopy, various sizes of endotracheal tubes (6.0, 7.0, and 8.0) with stylets, oropharyngeal airways, nasopharyngeal airways, and bougie.
- Difficult airway equipment may include a video laryngoscope (such as a C-Mac or GlideScope), a fiber optic bronchoscope, and an emergency cricothyroidotomy kit.
- The anesthesiologist may consider moving the patient to the operating room for a more controlled environment and easier access to equipment. This would include an anesthesia ventilator, an anesthesia cart, and easier access to an anesthesia technician and surgical technician.

(f) The intubation will be challenging:

- The learner should perform a rapid sequence induction with consideration for the use of cricoid pressure to reduce aspiration risk and manual cervical spine in-line stabilization to minimize cervical spine trauma.
- The learner may elect to start with a direct laryngoscopy for their first intubation attempt. They will encounter a grade 4 view and be unable to intubate. In between intubation attempts, they will find it difficult to mask ventilate and desaturation will occur. The patient will require two-handed bag mask ventilation with an oral airway, then oxygen saturation will improve.
- Alternatively, the learner may elect to start with a video laryngoscopy for their first intubation attempt. They will encounter a grade 3 view with a very swollen epiglottis. They will be unable to pass an endotracheal tube (ETT), even a 6.0 cuffed ETT.
- Bag mask ventilation between attempts will become increasingly difficult even with two-handed mask ventilation and an oral airway. The patient will desaturate further.
- The anesthesiologist should progress down the difficult airway algorithm and insert a LMA. The anesthesiologist should notify the surgeons of difficult intubation and ask them to prepare for possible emergency cricothyroidotomy.
- With the insertion of the LMA, ventilation will improve and oxygen saturation will improve. The surgeons should prepare for an emergency surgical airway but not yet cut the neck at this point.

- The anesthesiologist should use the fiber optic bronchoscope to intubate through the LMA. They will obtain a grade 1 view but again encounter a very swollen glottic opening including the vocal cords, arytenoids, and epiglottis. They will be able to pass a 6.0 cuffed endotracheal tube successfully.

3. Phase 3: Ongoing resuscitation.
    (a) After intubation and initial fluid resuscitation in the trauma bay, the patient will be more hemodynamically stable.
    (b) The learners should recognize that it is time to move the patient from the trauma bay to the burn intensive care unit (BICU).
    (c) The scenario will end here.

1.7 Anesthesiology Scoring Rubric

Topic: Major burn patient in respiratory distress		Completed	Not completed
Participants:			
Evaluators:			
Score:			
Tasks		Completed	Not completed
Phase 1: Initial survey and resuscitation			
Evaluation and communication	Identify the team leader and communicate pertinent information about the patient so far (i.e., ABCDE and AMPLE).		
Management	Ensure that full monitors are in place (SpO_2, EKG, BP, and $ETCO_2$).		
	Administer 100% FiO_2.		
	Establish additional IV access (peripheral or central).		
	Ensure the arterial line is placed.		
	Begin fluid resuscitation (20–40 cc/kg bolus vs. initiating Parkland formula).		
	Ensure initial labs are drawn: CBC, CMP, coagulation panel, ABG, lactate, type and screen/type and cross, blood cultures, urine cultures, urinalysis, troponin level, and urine toxicology screen. Consider carbon monoxide levels.		
Phase 2: Airway management			
Evaluation and communication	Communicate with surgeons their concern for smoke inhalation and possible aspiration events and the need to secure the airway quickly.		
	May discuss moving the patient to the operating room (OR) for intubation for an anticipated difficult airway.		
	Notify surgeons of significant airway edema during initial intubation attempts.		
	Ask the surgeons to prepare for possible emergency cricothyroidotomy.		
	Continually update surgeons on the status of bag mask ventilation and intubation attempts.		

(continued)

Topic: Major burn patient in respiratory distress			
Management	Perform timely intubation.		
	Double check airway supplies for anticipation of difficult airway: MOMSAID, various size laryngoscopes, ETTs, LMAs, bougie, GlideScope/ fiber optic bronchoscope, and emergent cricothyroidotomy kit.		
	Perform rapid sequence induction (RSI) with cricoid pressure and C-spine stabilization.		
	Recognize difficult airway after initial attempt with direct laryngoscopy or video laryngoscopy.		
	Identify airway edema.		
	Identify increasingly difficult bag mask ventilation.		
	Follow the difficult airway algorithm: Identify the inability to mask and the inability to intubate.		
	Place LMA.		
	Intubate with fiberoptic bronchoscope (FOB) through LMA with smaller ETT.		
Phase 3: Ongoing resuscitation and disposition			
Evaluation and communication	Discuss the disposition plan with surgeons including when it is safe to move from trauma bay to burn ICU.		
Management	Transport the patient to the BICU for further management and care.		

Tension Pneumothorax During Laparoscopy

Caitlin Krol and Claire Sampankanpanich Soria

2.1 Level of Training

– Anesthesiology resident
– General surgery resident

2.2 Learning Objectives

1. Review the risks of laparoscopic abdominal surgery.
2. Discuss the signs and symptoms of an intraoperative tension pneumothorax.
3. Review the management of a tension pneumothorax.

2.3 Simulator Environment

1. Location: main operating room of a tertiary care center.
2. Manikin setup:
    (a) Age: adult.
    (b) Lines: 1 x 20 gauge peripheral intravenous (PIV) line in the arm.
    (c) Monitors: non-invasive blood pressure (NIBP) cuff, 5-lead electrocardiogram (EKG), pulse oximeter, temperature.
3. Medications available:
    (a) Fluids: normal saline, lactated ringers, albumin.
    (b) Sedatives/hypnotics: propofol, etomidate, ketamine, inhaled anesthetics.
    (c) Paralytics: succinylcholine, rocuronium.

C. Krol (✉) · C. S. Soria
University of California, San Diego, San Diego, CA, USA
e-mail: ckrol@health.ucsd.edu; cssoria@health.ucsd.edu

© The Author(s), under exclusive license to Springer Nature Switzerland AG 2024
C. S. Soria, P. Yao (eds.), *Anesthesiology Simulation*,
https://doi.org/10.1007/978-3-031-80228-7_2

   (d) Cardiac agents: epinephrine, phenylephrine, ephedrine, vasopressin, atropine, glycopyrrolate, esmolol, labetalol, nicardipine, dopamine.

   (e) Narcotics: midazolam, fentanyl, hydromorphone.

4. Equipment available:

   (a) Airway equipment: anesthesia machine (including circuit, mask, and suction), laryngoscope and cuffed endotracheal tube (ETTs) of various sizes, stylette, oral airway, nasal trumpet, laryngeal mask airway (LMA), bougie. GlideScope and fiber optic tower are available if asked for.

   (b) Monitors: pulse oximeter, blood pressure cuff, 5-lead EKG, end-tidal carbon dioxde ($ETCO_2$) monitor, temperature probe.

   (c) Lines: arterial line kit and transducer, central line kit, and PIV kits are available upon request.

   (d) Crash cart with defibrillator outside the room available upon request.

2.4 Actors

1. Surgeon
2. Anesthesiologist
3. Circulator nurse
4. Surgical scrub technician
5. Anesthesia technician

2.5 Case Narrative

1. Background:

   (a) You are the surgical and anesthesia team working in the main operating room. Your case is a laparoscopic repair of a paraoesophageal hernia with Nissen fundoplication.

2. Pre-operative information provided:

   (a) Patient history: 62-year-old man, 120 kilograms (kg), body mass index (BMI) 40, with hypertension (HTN), chronic obstructive pulmonary disease (COPD), longtime smoker of 50 pack-years who discontinued smoking cigarettes 1 week prior to surgery, type 2 diabetes mellitus, and severe gastroesophageal reflux disease (GERD). He has been seen in gastroenterology and surgery clinics for post-prandial epigastric pain, occasional post-prandial dyspnea, and regurgitation of food for the past 2 years. He has tried anti-reflux medications without relief. Computed tomography (CT) scan of the abdomen with oral contrast previously showed herniation of the stomach along with the gastroesophageal junction into the thoracic cavity. The patient was diagnosed with a large type III paraesophageal hernia and is now scheduled for laparoscopic repair with Nissen fundoplication.

(b) Medications: hydrochlorothiazide, losartan, albuterol as needed, budesonide/formoterol, metformin, omeprazole.

(c) Allergies: no known drug allergies.

(d) Surgeries: total knee replacement 5 years ago under general anesthesia, no anesthetic complications.

(e) Labs: white blood cell (WBC) count 12, hemoglobin (Hb) 16, hematocrit (Hct) 48, platelets (Plt) 300, sodium (Na) 142, potassium (K) 3.8, chloride (Cl) 109, creatinine (Cr) 1.3, blood urea nitrogen (BUN) 18, glucose 130. Type and screen sample sent pre-operatively.

(f) Images:
- CT abdomen as described above.
- Chest X-ray (CXR): retrocardiac air-fluid level, some flattening of the diaphragm.

(g) Cardiac workup:
- EKG: rate of 70 beats per minute (bpm), normal sinus rhythm, rightward deviation of the P wave and QRS axis, low voltage QRS complexes in precordial leads, right atrial enlargement, and right ventricular hypertrophy.
- Transthoracic echocardiogram (TTE): left ventricular ejection fraction (LVEF) 53%, moderate tricuspid regurgitation, moderate pulmonary HTN with systolic pulmonary artery pressure of 50 mmHg, right atrial enlargement, moderate right ventricle hypertrophy, and mild–moderate left ventricle hypertrophy.

(h) Physical exam:
- General: obese man, sitting up in bed, awake, alert, oriented.
- Cardiac: regular rate and rhythm, a systolic murmur heard at the right sternal border.
- Respiratory: bilateral end-expiratory wheezing and a productive cough which the patient reports is all at his baseline.
- Abdominal: chronic reflux worse with lying flat, abdomen soft and non-tender to palpation, normal bowel sounds throughout.
- Neurologic: grossly normal strength and sensation in all four extremities.
- Airway: Mallampati IV, thick neck circumference with excess soft tissue around the neck and jaw, normal mouth opening, normal thyromental distance, normal neck range of motion, dentition intact.

2.6 Scenario Development

1. Phase 1: Induction and intubation
    (a) Pre-medication
    - The anesthesiologist learner may opt not to administer midazolam, given the patient's baseline moderate pulmonary HTN. Sedatives such as midazolam may cause respiratory depression, causing hypercarbia, acidosis,

increased pulmonary vascular resistance, and exacerbation of underlying pulmonary HTN. Alternatively, the anesthesiologist may opt to cautiously administer midazolam to alleviate patient anxiety but maintain close observation of the patient.

- The anesthesiologist may pre-medicate the patient with antiemetics or acid-reducing agents, such as sodium bicarbonate, famotidine, and metoclopramide, to decrease the risk of aspiration.
- The anesthesiologist may treat the patient's baseline COPD with an albuterol inhaler or albuterol nebulizer prior to induction to minimize the risk of bronchospasm with intubation.

(b) Induction and intubation

- The anesthesiologist may perform a rapid sequence induction.
- Intubation will proceed uneventfully. The patient will be easy to bag mask ventilate and easy to intubate by direct laryngoscopy.
- Vital signs will remain stable and within normal limits assuming the anesthesiologist anticipates and quickly preempts or treats hypotension expected with induction.
  - The anesthesiologist may choose a hypnotic agent that causes less myocardial depression such as etomidate or possibly ketamine, or may cautiously induce with propofol, and some combination of narcotics such as fentanyl.
  - The anesthesiologist may start a vasopressor or inotrope as a bolus or infusion prior to, during, or after induction.

(c) Additional lines

- The anesthesiologist should place an arterial line post-induction given the patient's cardiac status and location of surgery within the thorax.
- The anesthesiologist should also establish additional large-bore IV access.
- It will be easy to obtain PIV and arterial line access.

2. Phase 2: Difficulty ventilating and hemodynamic instability

(a) The surgeons will begin the case. The surgery will proceed uneventfully initially. The vital signs will be stable and within normal limits. The surgeons will be easily able to insert the ports and insufflate.

(b) While working on the para-esophageal herniation, the surgeons will encounter challenging anatomy and have difficulty grasping and positioning the hernia.

(c) The following will occur with the anesthesiologist's ventilator, assuming the learner had programmed the ventilator to volume-controlled ventilation (VCV) mode:

- The ventilator will alarm with a "high peak pressure" notification.
- Peak pressure will be >40 cmH2O.
- The ventilator will alarm with "tidal volumes unable to be achieved."
- Tidal volume delivered will be <200 cc, regardless of the set tidal volume.
- The $ETCO_2$ will decrease.

    (d) If the learner had programmed the ventilator to pressure-controlled ventilation (PCV), the following will occur with the ventilator:

- Tidal volume for a set peak pressure will decline to 200 cc, regardless of the set driving pressure and peak pressure.
- The ventilator will not alarm. The learner will need to check the ventilator settings and notice an acute drop in tidal volume.
- The $ETCO_2$ will decrease.

    (e) The following will occur with the monitors:

- The oxygen saturation will drop acutely.
- The heart rate will increase or decrease. The instructor may decide to make the patient tachycardic or bradycardic. Either can occur with tension pneumothorax.
- The blood pressure will decrease.

3. Phase 3: Recognition of tension pneumothorax and consideration of alternative differential diagnoses

    (a) The anesthesiologist should immediately notify the surgeons of acute, profound hemodynamic instability and difficulty ventilating.

    (b) The surgeons should survey their surgical field to identify a surgical cause.

- Surgical differential diagnoses may include:
  - Tension pneumothorax.
  - Tension hemothorax.
  - Venous air embolism.
  - Hemorrhage.
- During the survey, the surgeons will notice a large tear in the diaphragm.
  - The surgeons should decide how long it will take time to surgically repair the diaphragmatic tear. This should be weighed against how poorly the patient is doing hemodynamically and ventilation-wise. The surgeons may decide the patient is too unstable to tolerate the repair without an interim chest tube.

    (c) Tension pneumothorax should be high on the surgeon's differential.

- The surgeon therefore should move to desufflate the abdomen to prevent further expansion of the tension pneumothorax.
- The surgeon should remain in close communication with the anesthesiologist while they provide supportive measures to the patient.
- The surgeon should ask the circulator nurse and scrub tech for a chest tube STAT and consider emergently placing a chest tube to relieve the tension pneumothorax if the patient does not respond to supportive measures.

    (d) The anesthesiologists should simultaneously diagnose and treat.

- Initial treatment should include:
  - Opening all fluids wide open or manually hand bolusing the patient to try to improve preload and cardiac output.

- Administering inotropes and vasopressors as boluses and/or infusions. This may include: phenylephrine, ephedrine, epinephrine, dopamine, vasopressin, and atropine, which are often readily available in most anesthesia pharmacy carts.
- Switching to 100% FiO_2 and possibly hand bagging the patient to assess changes in compliance as the tension pneumothorax expands. The anesthesiologist will find that there is poor compliance and it is difficult to ventilate the patient due to high resistance.
- Consider discontinuing or decreasing volatile anesthetic in the setting of declining cardiac output.
- Recognizing that if this is a tension pneumothorax, it is primarily supportive measures, but that the patient may require decompression of the tension pneumothorax via (1) emergency needle decompression or (2) emergency chest tube insertion.
- If they have not done so already, the anesthesiologist should ask the surgeon to call for a chest tube and prepare for emergency chest tube insertion.
- Calling for help such as an anesthesia STAT to get more providers in the room.
- Calling for a crash cart to be brought to the room.
- The anesthesiologist may rule out other differential diagnoses by checking their ventilator programming, their circuit, and passing a soft suction catheter or fiber optic bronchoscope to examine the trachea-bronchial tree. All of this will be normal and functional.
- Differential diagnoses the anesthesiologist should consider include:
  - Tension pneumothorax.
  - Bronchospasm due to COPD exacerbation or anaphylaxis.
  - Mechanical obstruction such as ventilator malfunction, obstruction/ kinking/disconnection in the circuit, mucus plugging, or other obstruction in the endotracheal tube.
  - Tension hemothorax.
  - Venous air embolism.
  - Pulmonary embolism.
  - Myocardial infarction.
  - Hemorrhage.

4. Phase 4: Cardiac arrest
   (a) If the surgery and anesthesia teams do not move to place a chest tube, regardless of attempts at surgical repair and ongoing resuscitation medications administered so far in the scenario, the patient will devolve into cardiac arrest: ventricular tachycardia without a pulse.

(b) The learners should initiate Advanced Cardiac Life Support (ACLS), call for an anesthesia STAT if they have not done so already, and call for the crash cart. Initial ACLS next steps should include:
- Initiating chest compressions.
- Administering epinephrine 1 mg.
- Performing an unsynchronized cardioversion.

(c) With appropriate ACLS steps, the patient will convert from ventricular tachycardia without a pulse to normal sinus rhythm with a weak but palpable pulse.

(d) The learners should have recognized by now that tension pneumothorax is the most likely differential diagnosis. They should decompress the tension pneumothorax emergently:
- The anesthesiologist may perform an emergency needle decompression, such as insertion of a 14 G needle into the second intercostal space, midclavicular line, above the rib to avoid the neurovascular bundle.
  - Upon doing so, an audible sound of the rush of air being released will be heard.
  - The patient's ventilation and hemodynamics will start to improve.
- If they have not done so already, the surgeon should place an emergency chest tube. They will be able to do this easily.
  - Upon doing so, an audible sound of the rush of air being released will be heard.
  - The patient's ventilation and hemodynamics will improve substantially.
- The surgeon and anesthesiologist may call a radiology technician to take the chest X-ray intraoperatively to confirm chest tube placement and resolution of the pneumothorax.

5. Phase 5: Disposition
   (a) The anesthesia and surgical team will need to decide if they continue the surgery once the patient stabilizes.
   (b) The anesthesia team will need to decide if it is safe to extubate the patient.
   (c) Regardless, the patient should be transported to the intensive care unit (ICU) for observation post-operatively.

2.7   Anesthesiology Scoring Rubric

Topic: Tension pneumothorax		Completed	Not completed
Participants:			
Evaluators:			
Score:			
Tasks		Completed	Not completed
Phase 1: Induction and intubation			
Evaluation and communication	Discuss with surgeons the plan to establish additional IV access and arterial line post-induction.		
Management	Perform rapid sequence induction.		
	Establish additional IV access.		
	Place arterial line.		
Phase 2: Insufflation, difficulty ventilating, hemodynamic instability			
Evaluation and communication	Notify surgeons of sudden difficulty ventilating the patient.		
	Notify surgeons of sudden hemodynamic instability.		
Management	Survey ventilator settings and identify a drop in tidal volume for a given pressure.		
	Manually bag patient to identify poor compliance.		
	Perform a systematic sweep including checking the ventilator circuit for disconnections/obstructions, passing a soft suction catheter or fiber optic bronchoscope to survey the trachea-bronchial tree, auscultate lung fields, and survey the surgical field.		
	Survey monitors and identify arrhythmia and hypotension.		
	Identify possible differential diagnoses, recognizing tension pneumothorax or bronchospasm are the most likely causes.		
	Switch to 100% FiO_2.		
	Treat the hypotension and arrhythmia with pressors, inotropes, and/or fluid bolus.		
Phase 3: Tension pneumothorax			
Evaluation and communication	Notify surgeons of high suspicion for tension pneumothorax.		
	Ask the surgeons to desufflate the abdomen.		
	Ask the surgeons to consider inserting a chest tube.		
	Notify surgeons of the plan to perform emergency needle decompression.		
Management	Continue supportive measures: fluids, pressors, inotropes, and 100% FiO_2.		
	Call for the crash cart to be brought to room.		
	Call for help such as anesthesia STAT.		
	Perform emergent needle decompression with an appropriate-sized catheter and insertion site.		

(continued)

Topic: Tension pneumothorax			
Phase 4: Cardiac arrest			
Evaluation and communication	Notify surgeons that the patient is in cardiac arrest with a rhythm being ventricular tachycardia without a pulse.		
	Ask surgeons to start chest compressions immediately.		
Management	Initiate ACLS, including: Chest compressions Epinephrine 1 mg IV Unsynchronized cardioversion		
	If not done prior to cardiac arrest, perform emergent needle decompression.		
	If not done prior to cardiac arrest, ensure surgeons place chest tube.		
	Order the chest X-ray to confirm chest tube placement.		
Phase 5: Disposition			
Evaluation and communication	Discuss with surgeons whether to continue or abort surgery.		
	Discuss with surgeons whether to extubate in the operating room (OR) or go intubated to the ICU.		
Management	Transport to ICU for further management and care.		

Hemorrhagic Shock in Trauma (Stab Wound)

3

Scott Lewis, Graham Spurzem, Bryan Sandler, and Claire Sampankanpanich Soria

3.1 Level of Training

- Anesthesiology resident
- General surgery resident

3.2 Learning Objectives for Anesthesiology Residents

1. Review operating room management of acute, traumatic hemorrhagic shock.
2. Discuss how to optimize safety of induction of anesthesia in a patient in hemorrhagic shock.
3. Review massive transfusion protocol.

3.3 Learning Objectives for Surgery Residents

1. Review surgical approaches for management of acute, traumatic hemorrhagic shock due to intra-abdominal bleeding.
2. Review and perform 4-quadrant abdominal packing for control and identification of bleeding source.
3. Characterize the severity of visceral injury and determine appropriate management.
4. Control bleeding with appropriate needle and suture selection and suture technique.
5. Effectively communicate with the anesthesia team regarding identification and repair of injury and postoperative care.

S. Lewis (✉) · G. Spurzem · B. Sandler · C. S. Soria
University of California, San Diego, San Diego, CA, USA
e-mail: sjlewis@health.ucsd.edu; gspurzem@health.ucsd.edu; bsandler@health.ucsd.edu; cssoria@health.ucsd.edu

© The Author(s), under exclusive license to Springer Nature Switzerland AG 2024
C. S. Soria, P. Yao (eds.), *Anesthesiology Simulation*,
https://doi.org/10.1007/978-3-031-80228-7_3

3.4   Simulator Environment

1. Location: main operating room of a Level 1 trauma center.
2. Pig setup:
    (a) Age: adult.
    (b) Lines: 1 x intraosseous line in the uninjured leg.
    (c) Monitors: non-invasive blood pressure (NIBP) cuff, 5-lead electrocardiogram (EKG), and pulse oximeter (SpO_2).
3. Medications available:
    (a) Fluids: normal saline, lactated ringers, 5% albumin.
    (b) Blood products: massive transfusion protocol has been activated; blood products are en route to the operating room at the start of the case.
    (c) Sedatives/hypnotics: propofol, etomidate, ketamine, and inhaled anesthetics.
    (d) Paralytics: succinylcholine, rocuronium.
    (e) Cardiac agents: epinephrine, phenylephrine, ephedrine, atropine, glycopyrrolate, esmolol, labetalol, nicardipine, dopamine, and norepinephrine.
    (f) Narcotics: midazolam, fentanyl, and hydromorphone.
4. Equipment available:
    (a) Airway equipment: anesthesia machine (including circuit, mask, suction), laryngoscope and cuffed endotracheal tubes of various sizes, stylet, oropharyngeal airway, nasopharyngeal trumpet, laryngeal mask airway (LMA), and bougie. Video laryngoscope such as GlideScope or C-Mac and fiber optic bronchoscope are available upon request.
    (b) Monitors: non-invasive blood pressure (NIBP) cuff, 5-lead electrocardiogram (EKG), pulse oximeter (SpO_2), end-tidal carbon dioxide ($ETCO_2$), and temperature.
    (c) Lines: arterial line kit and transducer, central line kit, peripheral intravenous (PIV) kits, and Belmont or Rapid Infuser are all available upon request.
    (d) Crash cart with defibrillator is located outside the room and available upon request.
    (e) Ultrasound is available upon request.

3.5   Actors

1. Emergency medical technician.
2. Surgeon.
3. Anesthesiologist.
4. Anesthesia technician.
5. Circulator nurse.
6. Surgical scrub technician.

3.6   Case Narrative

1. Background:
   (a) You are the anesthesia and surgical teams on call overnight at a Level 1 trauma center.
2. You are the anesthesiologist team and surgical team on call at a Level 1 trauma center. You are paged STAT to the Trauma Resuscitation Operating Room for a Level 1 patient who is coming direct from the ambulance bay to the operating room.
3. Case scenario:
   (a) Report from emergency medical technicians:
       - Responded to call for a young man stabbed with a knife during a bar fight.
       - 30-year-old male with bruising to the eye, a bloody nose, cuts to both hands, and a single stab wound to the right upper quadrant of the abdomen.
       - Initial vital signs: HR 115, BP 80/50, Sat 100% on room air, temperature 36 °C, RR 20. Appears to be 6′, 80 kg, BMI 24.
       - Received 1 L crystalloid in the field via his intraosseous line.
       - The patient is screaming in pain. He denies using any alcohol or recreational drugs, but he smells of alcohol and marijuana. Patient denies any past medical history, allergies, medications, or surgical history.
   (b) Physical exam/Trauma Survey:
       - *Neuro*: extra-ocular movements intact (not cooperative), pupils equal/round/reactive to light, Glasgow Coma Scale (GCS) score of 13 (Eye 4, Verbal 4, Motor 5), appears acutely intoxicated.
       - *Cardiovascular*: tachycardic, no murmurs, and no rub.
       - *Respiratory*: spontaneously breathing on room air, breath sounds clear to auscultation bilaterally, and screaming loudly in pain.
       - *Abdomen*: rigid, distended, single stab round to RUQ with moderate oozing.
       - *Back*: atraumatic.
       - *Extremities*: weakly palpable distal pulses.

3.7   Scenario Development

1. Phase 1: Initial survey and pre-induction planning
   (a) The learners should identify a team leader and delegate tasks efficiently and effectively.
       - The surgeon should be the team leader in the operating room (OR).

  (b) The team leader should perform a rapid ABCDE assessment and brief history (consider AMPLE).
- ABCDE: Airway, Breathing, Circulation, Disability, Exposure.
- AMPLE: Allergies, Medications, Past medical history, Last oral intake, Events leading to Present Illness or Injury.

  (c) The team, hereafter defined as the surgeon and anesthesiologist, should ensure full monitors on the patient, including: 5-lead electrocardiogram (EKG), non-invasive blood pressure (NIBP) cuff, pulse oximeter (SpO_2), and end-tidal carbon dioxide ($ETCO_2$).

  (d) The anesthesiologist should place supplemental oxygen on the patient, such as a full face mask from the ventilator circuit to deliver 100% FiO_2 and monitor $ETCO_2$.

  (e) The team should verify with each other and the staff members present that the massive transfusion protocol (MTP) has been initiated and that blood products are en route to the OR.

  (f) Prior to induction, the team should discuss the patient's current hemodynamic state and the risk of bleeding once the tourniquet is removed.

  (g) The surgeon may ask the anesthesiologist to delay induction and intubation if the risk of bleeding is high. The anesthesiologist should resuscitate the patient with fluids, blood transfusion, and pressors as much as possible prior to induction.

2. Phase 2: Pre-induction resuscitation

  (a) The team should obtain additional large bore intravascular (IV) access. This may be: peripheral intravenous (PIVs), central line.

  (b) The team should consider placing an arterial line prior to induction to send off labs and more closely monitor hemodynamic instability during induction.

  (c) While obtaining vascular access, the team should draw a rainbow panel of labs, including: complete blood count (CBC), complete metabolic panel (CMP), lactate, coagulation panel, type and screen/type and cross, and urine toxicology screen.

  (d) The team should discuss when it is safe to induce and intubate the patient. Preferably, the team should resuscitate the patient first and evaluate the stab wound prior to induction to minimize hemodynamic collapse.

  (e) After obtaining access, initial resuscitation should include one or more of the following:
- Administering a fluid bolus (e.g., 20–40 cc/kg of crystalloid or 10–15 cc/kg of colloid).
- Transfusing packed red blood cells (if available).
- Starting an inotrope or vasopressor.

  (f) The team should perform imaging studies, including chest X-ray (CXR), and consider focused assessment of sonography in trauma (FAST) exam.
- FAST exam will be negative.
- CXR will be negative.

3. Phase 3: Induction of anesthesia
   (a) With the above measures, the patient's hypotension and tachycardia will improve.
   (b) The team should review the patient's current resuscitation status and agree whether it is ok to induce.
   (c) The anesthesiologist should perform a rapid sequence induction and intubation. Intubation will proceed uneventfully.
4. Phase 4: Decompensation after laparotomy
   (a) The surgeon should instruct the scrub nurse how to prep the patient and confirm that they have the instruments available for the procedure planned.
   (b) The surgeon should then proceed with an exploratory laparotomy.
       - At laparotomy:
       - There will be large volume, rapid bleeding from a liver laceration.
       - Patient's vital signs will acutely worsen to BP 60s/40s, HR 130s.
   (c) The anesthesiologist should alert the surgeon that the patient is becoming hemodynamically unstable.
   (d) The anesthesiologist should continue the resuscitation: massive transfusion in a balanced ratio (packed red blood cells, fresh frozen plasma, and platelets), crystalloids and colloids, and inotropes and pressors.
   (e) The anesthesiologist should send frequent arterial blood gases (ABGs) to evaluate the status of resuscitation, including metabolic acidosis, anemia, hypocalcemia, and hyperkalemia.
5. Phase 5: Repair of liver laceration and disposition
   (a) The surgeons should first perform 4-quadrant abdominal packing to identify the bleeding source and allow time for resuscitation.
   (b) The surgeons will be able to repair the liver laceration with electrocautery and simple hepatorrhaphy. The surgeon should repair the laceration with the appropriate needle and suture type.
   (c) Once the patient has stabilized and surgical hemostasis has been achieved, the surgeons and anesthesiologists should recap the events and current state of the resuscitation. This will include hemodynamic stability, recent labs (e.g., worsening versus improving anemia, thrombocytopenia, or metabolic acidosis).
   (d) The surgeons and anesthesiologists should discuss disposition course. They will likely decide to keep the patient intubated and transport to surgical intensive care unit (SICU) postoperatively for close observation and continued resuscitation.

3.8 Anesthesiology Scoring Rubric

Topic: Hemorrhagic shock due to stab wound			
Participants:			
Evaluators:			
Score:			
Tasks		Completed	Not completed
Phase 1: Initial survey and pre-induction planning			
Communication	Identify a team leader.		
	Clearly delegate tasks.		
	Confirm with surgeon/nurse that massive transfusion protocol was initiated.		
	Confirm with nurse that blood products are en route to the OR.		
	Prior to induction: Discuss with the surgeon the status of resuscitation, hemodynamic instability, and potential for bleed after tourniquet removal.		
	Work with the surgeon to resuscitate the patient as much as possible prior to induction.		
Phase 2: Pre-induction resuscitation			
Medical management	Place full monitors.		
	Place supplemental oxygen.		
	Establish large bore PIV or central line access.		
	Place arterial line prior to induction.		
	Administer fluid bolus of crystalloid and/or colloid.		
	Initiate inotropes/vasopressors.		
	Once blood products arrive: Transfuse in balanced ratio PRBCs, FFP, and Plts.		
	Send rainbow labs: ABG, CBC, BMP, coags, type and cross, UTox.		
Phase 3: Induction of anesthesia			
Evaluation and communication	Communicate with surgeons when pre-induction resuscitation is adequate and ready for induction.		
Management	Perform rapid sequence induction and intubation.		
Phase 4: Decompensation after tourniquet removal			
Evaluation and communication	Notify the surgeons that the patient is becoming hemodynamically unstable.		
Management	Escalate fluid resuscitation and uptitrate pressors.		
	Continue transfusing blood products: PRBCs, FFP, and/or platelets in a balanced ratio.		
	Obtain frequent ABGs to guide resuscitation.		
	May send repeat labs, including: Coagulation panel, TEG, and lactate.		
Phase 5: Disposition			
Evaluation and communication	Debrief with surgeons: Current hemodynamic stability, EBL, most recent labs, products given, status of resuscitation.		
	Discuss disposition planning, including whether to remain intubated.		
Management	Transport to ICU for further evaluation and care.		

3.9   Surgery Scoring Rubric

Topic: Hemorrhagic shock due to stab wound		Completed	Not completed
Participants:			
Evaluators:			
Score:			
Tasks			
Phase 1: Initial survey and pre-induction planning			
Communication	Identify a team leader.		
	Clearly delegate tasks.		
	Confirm with anesthesia/nurse that the massive transfusion protocol was initiated.		
	Confirm with the nurse that blood products are en route to the OR.		
	Prior to induction: Discuss with the anesthesia team the status of resuscitation and hemodynamic instability.		
	Work with the anesthesia team to resuscitate the patient as much as possible prior to induction.		
Phase 2: Pre-induction resuscitation and Phase 3: Induction of anesthesia—to be completed by the anesthesia team			
Phase 4: Decompensation after laparotomy			
Evaluation and communication	Notify the anesthesia team that there is a large amount of blood in the abdomen on initial inspection.		
Management	Perform 4-quadrant abdominal packing and evacuate blood.		
	Identify the liver injury and notify the anesthesia team.		
	Exclude other sources of bleeding (run the bowel, check other organs, and major vessels).		
	Assess the severity of liver laceration and determine appropriate management (i.e., suture repair).		
	Appropriate needle, suture, and repair technique selection (absorbable suture [e.g., 0 chromic] on blunt tip needle, horizontal mattress/figure of 8/simple suture).		
	Achieve hemostasis.		
Phase 5: Disposition			
Evaluation and communication	Debrief with anesthesia: Current hemodynamic stability, EBL, most recent labs, products given, status of resuscitation.		
	Discuss disposition planning including whether to remain intubated.		
Management	Transport to ICU for further evaluation and care.		

Hemorrhagic Shock in Trauma (IVC Tear)

4

Caitlin Krol, Graham Spurzem, Bryan Sandler,
and Claire Sampankanpanich Soria

4.1 Level of Training

– Anesthesiology resident
– General surgery resident

4.2 Learning Objectives for Anesthesiology Residents

1. Identify the surgical and anesthetic risk factors for laparoscopic surgery.
2. Discuss how to diagnose and manage surgical hemorrhage from surgical and anesthesia points of view.
3. Review classification and management of hemorrhagic shock.

4.3 Learning Objectives for Surgery Residents

1. Review surgical approaches for management of acute, traumatic hemorrhagic shock due to intra-abdominal bleeding.
2. Review the indications for converting from laparoscopic to open surgery.
3. Review and perform 4-quadrant abdominal packing for control and identification of bleeding source.
4. Control bleeding from major vessels with appropriate needle/suture selection and suture technique.
5. Correctly perform a small bowel resection.

C. Krol (✉) · G. Spurzem · B. Sandler · C. S. Soria
University of California, San Diego, San Diego, CA, USA
e-mail: ckrol@health.ucsd.edu; gspurzem@health.ucsd.edu;
bsandler@health.ucsd.edu; cssoria@health.ucsd.edu

C. S. Soria, P. Yao (eds.), *Anesthesiology Simulation*,
https://doi.org/10.1007/978-3-031-80228-7_4

6. Effectively communicate with the anesthesia team regarding identification and repair of injury and postoperative care.

4.4 Simulator Environment

1. Location: main operating room at a level 1 trauma center.
2. Pig setup:
   (a) Age: adult.
   (b) Lines: 1×18 gauge (G) peripheral intravenous (PIV) in the hand.
   (c) Monitors: non-invasive blood pressure (NIBP) cuff, 5-lead electrocardiogram (EKG), pulse oximeter, temperature probe.
3. Medications available:
   (a) Fluids: normal saline, lactated ringers, 5% albumin.
   (b) Blood products: 2 units of packed red blood cells (PRBCs).
   (c) Sedatives/hypnotics: propofol, etomidate, ketamine, inhaled anesthetics.
   (d) Paralytics: succinylcholine, rocuronium.
   (e) Cardiac agents: epinephrine, phenylephrine, ephedrine, vasopressin, atropine, glycopyrrolate, esmolol, labetalol, nicardipine, dopamine.
   (f) Narcotics: midazolam, fentanyl, hydromorphone.
4. Equipment available:
   (a) Airway equipment: anesthesia ventilator (including circuit, mask, and suction), laryngoscope, and cuffed endotracheal tubes (ETTs) of various sizes, stylet, oropharyngeal airway, nasopharyngeal airway, laryngeal mask airway (LMA), bougie. Video laryngoscope and fiberoptic bronchoscope are available if specifically requested by the learner.
   (b) Monitors: pulse oximeter, blood pressure cuff, 5-lead EKG, end-tidal carbon dioxide ($ETCO_2$) monitor. Additional monitors such as arterial line transducer, central venous pressure (CVP) transducer, and trans-esophageal echocardiogram (TEE) are available if specifically requested by the learner.
   (c) Lines: arterial line kit, central line kit including triple lumen and Cordis, PIV kits available upon request.
   (d) Crash cart with a defibrillator is outside the room and available upon request.

4.5 Actors

1. Surgeon
2. Anesthesiologist
3. Circulator nurse
4. Surgical scrub technician
5. Anesthesia technician

4.6   Case Narrative

1. Scenario background given to participants
   (a) You are the surgical and anesthesia team on trauma call at a level 1 trauma center.
   (b) The anesthesiologist learner will be waiting outside the room and will receive a page that says "level 1 diagnostic laparoscopy, peds vs. auto" (for "pedestrian versus automobile").
   (c) The surgeon learner in the scenario will be provided with extra information.
2. Additional information is to be given to the surgeon learner only. Please note: this information should be given only to the learners who are playing the role of trauma surgeons in the scenario. The learners who are playing the role of anesthesiologists will not be automatically given this information. It will be part of the communication aspect of this joint simulation scenario. The surgeon learners should communicate this critical information to the anesthesiologist learners. The anesthesiologist learners should also seek this information out. Methods may include review of the electronic medical records, sending an extra anesthesiologist to the trauma bay, and calling/paging/finding a surgeon in person to obtain this additional information.
   (a) Chief complaint: A 50-year-old woman who was walking her dog to the mailbox when a drunk driver jumped the curve and crashed into her. The driver was speeding through a residential area. The patient did not lose consciousness but reports being thrown on the roof of the vehicle and onto the street. She has been having severe abdominal pain since then, and her abdomen feels distended.
   (b) Past medical history: hypertension, type 2 diabetes mellitus.
   (c) Medications: amlodipine, lisinopril, metformin.
   (d) Allergies: penicillin (hives).
   (e) Vital signs: 5′6″, 65 kg, BMI 23, heart rate (HR) 115 beats per minute (bpm), sinus tachycardia; pulse oximetry (SpO_2) 98% on room air, NIBP 80/50 mmHg, temperature (T) 36.5 °C.
      - Initial blood pressure on admission was 70/40 and improved to 80/50 after 1 L of lactated Ringer's bolus by emergency medical services (EMS) en route to the trauma bay.
   (f) Past surgical history: laparoscopic appendectomy at age 20 years old, laparoscopic ovarian cystectomy at age 40 years old for a dermoid cyst.
   (g) Labs: sodium (Na) 138, chloride (Cl) 108, potassium (K) 3.6, bicarbonate (HCO3) 24, blood urea nitrogen (BUN) 11, creatinine (Cr) 0.9, glucose 90, hemoglobin (Hb) 10, hematocrit (Hct) 30, platelets (Plt) 150, white blood cell (WBC) 14.
   (h) Imaging: chest x-ray in the trauma bay was negative (no fractures, no pleural effusion, no pneumothorax, no hemothorax, normal cardiac profile); focused assessment of sonography in trauma (FAST) exam was positive for free fluid in the abdomen.
   (i) Cardiac workup:

- 12-lead EKG: sinus tachycardia with T-wave inversions, rate of 119 bpm.
- Previously healthy, physically active, doing Zumba and jogging, no previous echocardiogram.

(j) Physical exam:
- General: anxious, well-nourished woman, awake, alert, oriented, moaning in pain, complaining that her abdomen hurts a lot.
- Cardiac: fast rate, regular rhythm, no murmurs/rubs/gallops.
- Pulmonary: clear to auscultation bilaterally.
- Abdominal: distended abdomen, tender to palpation.
- Neurologic: C-collar in place, appears grossly intact, moves all four extremities with equal strength but limited by pain.
- Skin: road rash, cuts, and bruises; no broken bones in the extremities noted.
- Airway: Mallampati II, normal thyromental distance, normal mouth opening, full neck range of motion, intact dentition.

4.7 Scenario Development

1. Phase 1: Preparation prior to induction
   (a) Surgical team
   - The surgeons should communicate with the scrub tech and circulator nurse, which surgical trays they need open now versus which should be available in the room or nearby in case they need to convert from laparoscopic to open.
   - The surgeons should communicate to the whole operating room team any relevant information about the patient's past medical history (PMH) and current illness. This includes an estimate of blood loss (EBL) so far, the current status of any resuscitation, the anticipated severity of bleeding, and the potential source of bleeding.
   - The surgeons may also discuss with the anesthesiologists' recommendations for vascular access and blood products to have in the room.
   (b) Anesthesia team
   - The anesthesiologists should seek additional information about the patient, including past medical history, history of present illness (HPI), current access, resuscitation measures implemented so far, recent labs, blood products available, current EBL, predicted additional blood loss, and source of bleed. They may try to find this information from the electronic medical record, send an available anesthesiologist to the trauma bay, and/or speak with the surgeon in person/by phone.
   - The anesthesiologists should communicate with the surgeons about recommendations or plans for additional access (e.g., large-bore PIV versus central line), invasive monitors (e.g., arterial line or CVP), and blood products. Depending on this discussion, the anesthesiologists may also prepare inotropes and pressors.

- The anesthesiologists should notify the surgeons that prior to induction and intubation, they will better resuscitate the patient with fluids and potentially pressors to offset the sympathectomy and hemodynamic instability that may occur with induction medications and initiation of positive pressure ventilation.
- The anesthesiologist should name a brief timeframe in which to achieve these tasks, understanding that the surgeons need to open the abdomen as soon as possible to identify and control the source of bleeding. Anesthesia tasks prior to induction should include:
  - Establishing large-bore upper extremity PIV access.
  - Placing an arterial line.
  - Administering a fluid bolus (e.g., 20–40 cc/kg of crystalloid or 10–15 cc/kg of colloid).
  - Possibly starting an inotrope or vasopressor.
- The surgeons may begin prepping the abdomen and positioning the abdomen in conjunction with the anesthesiologists performing these tasks to decrease the time to surgical incision.
- The patient's tachycardia and hypotension will improve with this initial resuscitation.

2. Phase 2: Induction, intubation, and start of diagnostic laparoscopy
   (a) Induction and intubation:
   - The anesthesiologist should communicate when they are ready for induction. The anesthesiologists should perform a rapid sequence induction.
   - Induction and intubation will proceed uneventfully. The airway will be secured easily. No aspiration will occur. The patient will sustain a small decline in blood pressure but remain within normal mean arterial pressures (MAPs).
   (b) Start of diagnostic laparoscopy:
   - The surgeons will insert ports and begin diagnostic laparoscopy. They will note that the abdomen appears to have a large amount of clotted blood, but there is no obvious source of bleeding.
   - The patient's vital signs will slowly start to worsen, with a slight increase in HR and a slight drop in blood pressure. The anesthesiologist will likely treat this with a fluid bolus and uptitration of pressors.
   - The surgeons may perform an irrigation and lavage to try to identify the source of bleeding but still not find anything alarming.

3. Phase 3: Hemodynamic instability and identification of inferior vena cava (IVC) tear
   (a) As the surgeons continue looking through the abdomen, such as running the bowel or moving aside some of the existing blood clots, they will unintentionally dislodge a clot that was tamponading the IVC. There is also a single destructive small bowel injury requiring resection.
   (b) The patient will quickly start hemorrhaging blood through the newly identified IVC tear and become increasingly tachycardic and hypotensive.

   (c) The surgeons should communicate this finding to the anesthesiologists. The anesthesiologists will escalate fluid resuscitation, initiate blood transfusion, and uptitrate pressors as needed.

   (d) The surgeons should also notify the scrub tech and circulator nurse and tell them they will emergently convert from laparoscopic to exploratory laparotomy.

   (e) The surgeons may try to report an estimated blood loss and ask the anesthesiologists to transfuse any number of PRBCs, fresh frozen plasma (FFP), and/or platelets (Plt).

   (f) The surgeons and anesthesiologists may also decide to initiate a massive transfusion protocol (MTP) to obtain additional blood products faster.

   (g) The surgeons and anesthesiologists should continually communicate with each other regarding the status of resuscitation (e.g., volume and amount of fluids, blood products, and pressors administered thus far from the anesthesiologists) and the current state of surgical hemostasis (e.g., estimated blood loss, rapidity of bleeding, how close to surgical hemostasis from the surgeons).

   (h) Anesthesiologists should send frequent arterial blood gas (ABG) samples to assess the status of their resuscitation. They may also send a thromboelastogram (TEG) and lactate. Initial ABG will show metabolic acidosis and anemia. With appropriate volume resuscitation and blood transfusion, this will improve.

4. Phase 4: Repair of IVC tear and disposition

   (a) The surgeons will perform an exploratory laparotomy and then 4-quadrant abdominal packing to identify the bleeding source and allow time for resuscitation.

   (b) The surgeons will be able to repair the IVC tear and perform a small bowel resection.

   (c) Once the patient has stabilized and surgical hemostasis has been achieved, the surgeons and anesthesiologists should recap the events and current state of the resuscitation. This will include hemodynamic stability and recent labs (e.g., worsening versus improving anemia, thrombocytopenia, or metabolic acidosis).

   (d) The surgeons and anesthesiologists should discuss the disposition course. They will likely decide to keep the patient intubated and transport them to the surgical intensive care unit (SICU) postoperatively for close observation and continued resuscitation.

   (e) The scenario will end here.

Anesthesiology Scoring Rubric

Topic: Hemorrhagic shock due to IVC tear		Completed	Not completed
Participants:			
Evaluators:			
Score:			
Tasks			
Phase 1: Preparation			
Evaluation and communication	Ask surgeons for additional information about the patient, including PMH, HPI, current vascular access, resuscitation measures implemented so far, recent labs, blood products available, current EBL, predicted additional blood loss, and source of bleed. Discuss with the surgeons the plan to establish additional access and volume resuscitate the patient prior to induction.		
Management	Establish large-bore PIV access prior to induction. Place arterial line prior to induction. Administer a fluid bolus and start inotropes/vasopressors prior to induction.		
Phase 2: Induction, intubation, and surgical start			
Evaluation and communication	Communicate with surgeons when pre-induction resuscitation is adequate and ready for induction. Ask the surgeons to hold manual cervical in-line stabilization during intubation.		
Management	Perform rapid sequence induction including C-spine stabilization.		
Phase 3: Hemorrhage			
Evaluation and communication	Notify the surgeons that the patient is becoming hemodynamically unstable.		
Management	Escalate fluid resuscitation and uptitrate pressors. Begin transfusing blood products: PRBCs, FFP, and/or platelets in a balanced ratio. Initiate massive transfusion protocol. Obtain frequent arterial blood gas to guide resuscitation. Send additional labs, including a coagulation panel, TEG, and lactate.		
Phase 4: Disposition			
Evaluation and communication	Debrief with surgeons: Current hemodynamic stability, EBL, most recent labs, products given, and status of resuscitation. Discuss disposition planning including whether to remain intubated.		
Management	Transport to ICU for further evaluation and care.		

Surgery Scoring Rubric

Topic: Hemorrhagic shock due to IVC tear		Completed	Not completed
Participants:			
Evaluators:			
Score:			
Tasks			
Phase 1: Preparation			
Evaluation and communication	Communicate with anesthesia regarding the following: PMH, HPI, current vascular access, resuscitation measures implemented so far, recent labs, blood products available, current EBL, predicted additional blood loss, and source of bleed.		
	Discuss with the anesthesia about plans to establish additional access and volume resuscitate the patient prior to induction.		
Phase 2: Induction, intubation, and surgical start to be completed by anesthesia			
Phase 3: Hemorrhage management			
Evaluation and communication	Notify anesthesia of IVC and small bowel injuries upon identification.		
Management	Obtain laparoscopic abdominal access and place ports.		
	Identify IVC and small bowel injuries.		
	Convert to open.		
	Perform 4-quadrant abdominal packing and evacuate blood.		
	Exclude other sources of bleeding and injuries (run the bowel, other major organs, and vessels. May identify small bowel injury at this time).		
	Assess the severity of IVC and small bowel injuries and determine appropriate management (i.e., suture repair of IVC and small bowel resection).		
	Appropriate needle, suture, and repair technique selection for IVC injury? (5-0/6-0 prolene on taper needle, running suture/figure of 8/simple interrupted).		
	Correctly perform stapled small bowel resection with appropriate suture, needle, and stapler.		
	Achieve hemostasis.		
Phase 4: Disposition			
Evaluation and communication	Debrief with anesthesia: Current hemodynamic stability, EBL, most recent labs, products given, and status of resuscitation.		
	Discuss disposition planning including whether to remain intubated.		
Management	Transport to ICU for further evaluation and care.		

Hemorrhagic Shock in Trauma (Solid Organ Injury)

5

Caitlin Krol, Graham Spurzem, Bryan Sandler,
and Claire Sampankanpanich Soria

5.1 Level of Training

– Anesthesiology resident
– General surgery resident

5.2 Learning Objectives for Anesthesiology Residents

1. Review operating room management of acute, traumatic hemorrhagic shock.
2. Discuss how to optimize safety of induction of anesthesia in a patient in hemorrhagic shock.
3. Review massive transfusion protocol.

5.3 Learning Objectives for Surgery Residents

1. Review surgical approaches for management of acute, traumatic hemorrhagic shock due to intra-abdominal bleeding.
2. Review and perform 4-quadrant abdominal packing for control and identification of bleeding source.
3. Characterize the severity of visceral injury and determine appropriate management.
4. Control bleeding with appropriate needle and suture selection and suture technique.
5. Effectively communicate with anesthesia team regarding identification and repair of injury and postoperative care.

C. Krol (✉) · G. Spurzem · B. Sandler · C. S. Soria
University of California, San Diego, San Diego, CA, USA
e-mail: ckrol@health.ucsd.edu; gspurzem@health.ucsd.edu; bsandler@health.ucsd.edu;
cssoria@health.ucsd.edu

5.4 Simulator Environment

1. Location: main operating room of a Level 1 trauma center.
2. Pig setup:
   (a) Age: adult.
   (b) Lines: 1 × intraosseous line in the leg.
   (c) Monitors: non-invasive blood pressure (NIBP) cuff, 5-lead electrocardiogram (EKG), and pulse oximeter (SpO_2).
3. Medications available:
   (a) Fluids: normal saline, lactated ringers, and 5% albumin.
   (b) Blood products: massive transfusion protocol has been activated; blood products are en route to the operating room at the start of the case.
   (c) Sedatives/hypnotics: propofol, etomidate, ketamine, and inhaled anesthetics.
   (d) Paralytics: succinylcholine and rocuronium.
   (e) Cardiac agents: epinephrine, phenylephrine, ephedrine, atropine, glycopyrrolate, esmolol, labetalol, nicardipine, dopamine, and norepinephrine.
   (f) Narcotics: midazolam, fentanyl, and hydromorphone.
4. Equipment available:
   (a) Airway equipment: anesthesia machine (including circuit, mask, suction), laryngoscope and cuffed endotracheal tubes of various sizes, stylet, oropharyngeal airway, nasopharyngeal trumpet, laryngeal mask airway (LMA), bougie. Video laryngoscopes such as GlideScope or C-Mac and fiberoptic bronchoscope are available upon request.
   (b) Monitors: non-invasive blood pressure (NIBP) cuff, 5-lead electrocardiogram (EKG), pulse oximeter (SpO_2), end-tidal carbon dioxide ($ETCO_2$), and temperature.
   (c) Lines: arterial line kit and transducer, central line kit, peripheral intravenous (PIV) kits, and Belmont or rapid infuser are all available upon request.
   (d) Crash cart with defibrillator is located outside the room and available upon request.
   (e) Ultrasound is available upon request.

5.5 Actors

1. Emergency medical technician.
2. Surgeon.
3. Anesthesiologist.
4. Anesthesia technician.
5. Circulator nurse.
6. Surgical scrub technician.

5.6   Case Narrative

1. Background:
   (a) You are the anesthesia and surgical teams on call overnight at a Level 1 trauma center.
       - You are the anesthesiologist team and surgical team on call at a level 1 trauma center. You are paged STAT to the Trauma Resuscitation Operating Room for a Level 1 patient who is coming direct from the ambulance bay to the operating room.
2. Case scenario:
   (a) Report from emergency medical technicians:
       - Responded to call for a young man hit by a car on a residential street.
       - 30-year-old male with bruising to the eye, a bloody nose, cuts to both hands, and a firm distended abdomen with bruising.
       - Initial vital signs: HR 115, BP 80/50, Sat 100% on room air, temperature 36 °C, RR 20. Appears to be 6′, 80 kg, BMI 24.
       - Received 1 L crystalloid in the field via his intraosseous line.
       - The patient is screaming in pain. He denies using any alcohol or recreational drugs. The patient denies any past medical history, allergies, medications, or surgical history.
   (b) Physical exam/trauma survey:
       - *Neuro*: GCS 15
       - *Cardiovascular*: tachycardic, no murmurs, no rub
       - *Respiratory*: spontaneously breathing on room air, breath sounds clear to auscultation bilaterally, screaming loudly in pain
       - *Abdomen*: rigid, distended, overlying bruising
       - *Back*: atraumatic
       - *Extremities*: weakly palpable distal pulses

5.7   Scenario Development

1. Phase 1: Initial survey and pre-induction planning
   (a) The learners should identify a team leader and delegate tasks efficiently and effectively.
       - The surgeon should be the team leader in the operating room (OR).
   (b) The team leader should perform a rapid ABCDE assessment and brief history (consider AMPLE).
       - ABCDE: Airway, Breathing, Circulation, Disability, Exposure.
       - AMPLE: Allergies, Medications, Past medical history, Last oral intake, Events leading to Present Illness or Injury.

(c) The team, hereafter defined as the surgeon and anesthesiologist, should be ensure full monitors on the patient, including: 5-lead electrocardiogram (EKG), non-invasive blood pressure (NIBP) cuff, pulse oximeter (SpO_2), and end-tidal carbon dioxide ($ETCO_2$).

(d) The anesthesiologist should place supplemental oxygen on the patient, such as a full face mask from the ventilator circuit to, deliver 100% FiO_2 and monitor $ETCO_2$.

(e) The team should verify with each other and the staff members present that the massive transfusion protocol (MTP) has been initiated and that blood products are en route to the OR.

(f) Prior to induction, the team should discuss the patient's current hemodynamic state and the risk of bleeding once the tourniquet is removed.

(g) The surgeon may ask the anesthesiologist to delay induction and intubation if the risk of bleeding is high. The anesthesiologist should resuscitate the patient with fluids, blood transfusion, and pressors as much as possible prior to induction.

2. Phase 2: Pre-induction resuscitation

(a) The team should obtain additional large bore intravascular (IV) access. This may be: peripheral intravenous (PIVs), central line.

(b) The team should consider placing an arterial line prior to induction to send off labs and more closely monitor hemodynamic instability during induction.

(c) While obtaining vascular access, the team should draw a rainbow panel of labs, including complete blood count (CBC), complete metabolic panel (CMP), lactate, coagulation panel, type and screen /type and cross, and urine toxicology screen.

(d) The team should discuss when it is safe to induce and intubate the patient. Preferably, the team should resuscitate the patient first and evaluate the stab wound prior to induction to minimize hemodynamic collapse.

(e) After obtaining access, initial resuscitation should include one or more of the following:
- Administering a fluid bolus (e.g., 20–40 cc/kg of crystalloid or 10–15 cc/kg of colloid).
- Transfusing packed red blood cells (if available).
- Starting an inotrope or vasopressor.

(f) The team should perform imaging studies, including chest X-ray (CXR) and consider focused assessment of sonography in trauma (FAST) exam.
- FAST exam will be negative.
- CXR will be negative.

3. Phase 3: Induction of anesthesia

(a) With the above measures, the patient's hypotension and tachycardia will improve.

   (b) The team should review the patient's current resuscitation status and agree whether it is ok to induce.

   (c) The anesthesiologist should perform a rapid sequence induction and intubation. Intubation will proceed uneventfully.

4. Phase 4: Decompensation after laparotomy

   (a) The surgeon should instruct the scrub nurse how to prep the patient and confirm that they have the instruments available for the procedure planned.

   (b) The surgeon should then proceed with an exploratory laparotomy.

   (c) At laparotomy:
- There will be large volume, rapid bleeding from a liver laceration, gallbladder laceration, and shattered spleen.
- Patient's vital signs will acutely worsen to BP 60s/40s, HR 130s.

   (d) The anesthesiologist should alert the surgeon that the patient is becoming hemodynamically unstable.

   (e) The anesthesiologist should continue the resuscitation: massive transfusion in a balanced ratio (packed red blood cells, fresh frozen plasma, and platelets), crystalloids and colloids, and inotropes and pressors.

   (f) The anesthesiologist should send frequent arterial blood gases (ABGs) to evaluate the status of resuscitation, including metabolic acidosis, anemia, hypocalcemia, and hyperkalemia.

5. Phase 5: Repair of liver laceration, cholecystectomy, splenectomy, and disposition

   (a) The surgeons should first perform 4-quadrant abdominal packing to identify the bleeding source and allow time for resuscitation.

   (b) The surgeons will be able to repair the liver laceration with electrocautery and simple hepatorrhaphy. The surgeon should repair the laceration with the appropriate needle and suture type. The gallbladder and spleen injuries require cholecystectomy and splenectomy, respectively.

   (c) Once the patient has stabilized and surgical hemostasis has been achieved, the surgeons and anesthesiologists should recap the events and the current state of the resuscitation. This will include hemodynamic stability, recent labs (e.g., worsening versus improving anemia, thrombocytopenia, or metabolic acidosis).

   (d) The surgeons and anesthesiologists should discuss the disposition course. They will likely decide to keep the patient intubated and transport to surgical intensive care unit (SICU) postoperatively for close observation and continued resuscitation.

5.8 Anesthesiology Scoring Rubric

Topic: Hemorrhagic shock due to solid organ injury			
Participants:			
Evaluators:			
Score:			
Tasks		Completed	Not completed
Phase 1: Initial survey and pre-induction planning			
Communication	Identify a team leader.		
	Clearly delegate tasks.		
	Confirm with surgeon/nurse that the massive transfusion protocol was initiated.		
	Confirm with the nurse that blood products are en route to the OR.		
	Prior to induction: Discuss with the surgeon the status of resuscitation, hemodynamic instability, and potential for bleed after tourniquet removal.		
	Work with the surgeon to resuscitate the patient as much as possible prior to induction.		
Phase 2: Pre-induction resuscitation			
Medical management	Place full monitors.		
	Place supplemental oxygen.		
	Establish large bore PIV or central line access.		
	Place arterial line prior to induction.		
	Administer fluid bolus of crystalloid and/or colloid.		
	Initiate inotropes/vasopressors.		
	Once blood products arrive: Transfuse in balanced ratio PRBCs, FFP, and Plts.		
	Send rainbow labs: ABG, CBC, BMP, coags, type and cross, UTox.		
Phase 3: Induction of anesthesia			
Evaluation and communication	Communicate with the surgeons when pre-induction resuscitation is adequate and ready for induction.		
Management	Perform rapid sequence induction and intubation.		
Phase 4: Decompensation after tourniquet removal			
Evaluation and communication	Notify the surgeons that the patient is becoming hemodynamically unstable.		
Management	Escalate fluid resuscitation and uptitrate pressors.		
	Continue transfusing blood products: PRBCs, FFP, and/or platelets in a balanced ratio.		
	Obtain frequent ABGs to guide resuscitation.		
	May send repeat labs, including: Coagulation panel, TEG, and lactate.		
Phase 5: Disposition			
Evaluation and communication	Debrief with surgeons: Current hemodynamic stability, EBL, most recent labs, products given, and status of resuscitation.		
	Discuss disposition planning, including whether to remain intubated.		
Management	Transport to ICU for further evaluation and care.		

5.9   Surgery Scoring Rubric

Topic: Hemorrhagic shock due to solid organ injury		Completed	Not completed
Participants:			
Evaluators:			
Score:			
Tasks		Completed	Not completed
Phase 1: Initial survey and pre-induction planning			
Communication	Identify a team leader.		
	Clearly delegate tasks.		
	Confirm with anesthesia/nurse that the massive transfusion protocol was initiated.		
	Confirm with the nurse that blood products are en route to the OR.		
	Prior to induction: Discuss with the anesthesia team the status of resuscitation and hemodynamic instability.		
	Work with the anesthesia team to resuscitate the patient as much as possible prior to induction.		
Phase 2: Pre-induction resuscitation and Phase 3: Induction of anesthesia—to be completed by anesthesia team			
Phase 4: Decompensation after laparotomy			
Evaluation and communication	Notify the anesthesia team that there is a large amount of blood in the abdomen on initial inspection.		
Management	Perform 4-quadrant abdominal packing and evacuate blood.		
	Identify the liver, gallbladder, and spleen injuries and notify the anesthesia team.		
	Exclude other sources of bleeding (run the bowel, check other organs and major vessels).		
	Assess the severity of liver laceration and determine appropriate management (i.e., suture repair).		
	Appropriate needle, suture, and repair technique selection for liver laceration (absorbable suture [e.g. 0 chromic] on blunt tip needle, horizontal mattress/figure of 8/simple suture).		
	Assess the severity of the gallbladder laceration and determine appropriate management (i.e., cholecystectomy).		
	Assess the severity of the spleen injury and determine appropriate management (i.e., splenectomy).		
	Achieve hemostasis.		
Phase 5: Disposition			
Evaluation and communication	Debrief with anesthesia: Current hemodynamic stability, EBL, most recent labs, products given, and status of resuscitation.		
	Discuss disposition planning including whether to remain intubated.		
Management	Transport to ICU for further evaluation and care.		

Malignant Hyperthermia

6

Claire Sampankanpanich Soria

6.1 Level of Training

– Anesthesiology resident
– General surgery resident

6.2 Learning Objectives

1. Describe the signs and symptoms of malignant hyperthermia (MH).
2. Discuss the management of MH.

6.3 Simulator Environment

1. Location: main operating room of a tertiary care medical center.
2. Manikin setup:
   (a) Age: adult.
   (b) Lines: 1 × 18 gauge (G) peripheral intravenous (PIV) in the hand.
   (c) Monitors: non-invasive blood pressure (NIBP) cuff, 5-lead electrocardiogram (EKG), pulse oximeter, temperature probe.
3. Medications available:
   (a) Fluids: normal saline, lactated ringers, 5% albumin.
   (b) Blood products: 2 units of packed red blood cells (PRBCs).
   (c) Sedatives/hypnotics: propofol, etomidate, ketamine, inhaled anesthetics.
   (d) Paralytics: succinylcholine, rocuronium.

C. S. Soria (✉)
University of California, San Diego, San Diego, CA, USA
e-mail: cssoria@health.ucsd.edu

© The Author(s), under exclusive license to Springer Nature Switzerland AG 2024
C. S. Soria, P. Yao (eds.), *Anesthesiology Simulation*,
https://doi.org/10.1007/978-3-031-80228-7_6

   (e) Cardiac agents: epinephrine, phenylephrine, ephedrine, vasopressin, atropine, glycopyrrolate, esmolol, labetalol, nicardipine, dopamine.
   (f) Additional medications: calcium chloride, insulin, sodium bicarbonate, dextrose, albuterol.
   (g) Narcotics: midazolam, fentanyl, hydromorphone.
4. Equipment available:
   (a) Airway equipment: anesthesia ventilator (including circuit, mask, and suction), laryngoscope and cuffed endotracheal tubes (ETTs) of various sizes, stylet, oropharyngeal airway, nasopharyngeal airway, laryngeal mask airway (LMA), bougie. Video laryngoscope and fiberoptic bronchoscope are available if specifically requested by the learner.
   (b) Monitors: pulse oximeter, blood pressure cuff, 5-lead EKG, end-tidal carbon dioxide ($ETCO_2$) monitor. Additional monitors such as arterial line transducer, central venous pressure (CVP) transducer, and trans-esophageal echocardiogram (TEE) are available if specifically requested by the learner.
   (c) Lines: arterial line kit, central line kit including triple lumen and Cordis, PIV kits available upon request.
   (d) Crash cart with a defibrillator is in the hallway and available upon request.
   (e) Malignant hyperthermia (MH) cart is in the hallway and basic metabolic panel (BMP), complete blood count (CBC), and creatine kinase (CK) labs are available upon request. This cart contains standard contents such as dantrolene (Ryanodex) formulation, sterile water, sodium bicarbonate, dextrose, calcium chloride, regular insulin, refrigerated cold saline solution, charcoal filters, and disposable cold packs.

6.4 Actors

1. Surgeon
2. Anesthesiologist
3. Circulator nurse
4. Surgical scrub technician
5. Anesthesia technician

6.5 Case Narrative

1. Scenario background given to participants:
   (a) You are the anesthesia and surgical team working at an outpatient surgical center.
   (b) The patient is a 25-year-old woman, 5′5″, 90 kg, BMI 33.3, with obesity and childhood asthma who is undergoing laparoscopic cholecystectomy for symptomatic cholelithiasis.
   (c) Past medical history: obesity; asthma as a child, never hospitalized, never intubated, has not required a rescue albuterol inhaler since she was a teenager.

(d) Medications: none.

(e) Allergies: none.

(f) Past surgical history: laparoscopic appendectomy for acute appendicitis when she was 9 years old.

(g) Labs: Hemoglobin 13.0, Hematocrit 39.0, Platelets 200K.

2. Phase 1: Induction

   (a) The anesthesia and surgery teams will perform a timeout prior to induction, confirming equipment, allergies, fire risk, correct patient, and site.

   (b) The anesthesiologist will perform a routine induction and intubation. This will be uneventful. The patient will be easy to intubate and will remain hemodynamically stable through induction.

   (c) The anesthesiologist may choose succinylcholine or rocuronium for a muscle relaxant for intubation. The anesthesiologist will likely maintain the patient on volatile anesthetic.

   (d) If the anesthesiologist chooses succinylcholine for intubation, the patient will have masseter muscle spasm, and it will be difficult to open the mouth for intubation. For the scenario, the anesthesiologist will be able to successfully intubate the patient by direct laryngoscopy though it will be challenging. The anesthesiologist may elect to convert to video laryngoscopy or fiberoptic bronchoscopy for intubation.

   (e) Regardless of the choice of paralytic for intubation, the patient will demonstrate an elevated $ETCO_2$ in the 50s shortly after being placed on the ventilator after intubation.

   (f) The anesthesiologist may increase the minute ventilation to lower the $ETCO_2$. The anesthesiologist will likely attribute this hypercarbia to the patient having been apneic during intubation time.

3. Phase 2: Abdomen insufflation and development of hypercarbia and hyperthermia

   (a) The surgeon will proceed with starting the surgery, including prepping the patient, positioning, inserting trocars, and beginning insufflation.

   (b) The patient's $ETCO_2$ will continue to rise to the 60s, 70s, and 80s, progressively worsening throughout the case. It will not decrease even as the anesthesiologist attempts to increase minute ventilation by increasing tidal volume and respiratory rate.

   (c) The patient's temperature will rise to 38, 39, 40, and 41 °C and will not lower until the anesthesiologist actively attempts to cool the patient.

   (d) The patient will develop muscle rigidity. The surgeon will notice that it is difficult to move their trocars. The surgeon may ask the anesthesiologist if the patient is light under anesthesia and if the patient has adequate muscle relaxation. If the anesthesiologist used rocuronium for intubation, the patient will have zero twitches on the peripheral nerve stimulator train of four tests.

4. Phase 3: Diagnosis of malignant hyperthermia

   (a) The anesthesiologist should notify the surgeon that the patient is increasingly hypercarbic and hyperthermic.

    (b) The anesthesiologist should ask the surgeon to pause surgery if possible so that they can investigate for suspected MH.

    (c) The surgeon should communicate with the anesthesiologist about where they are in the surgery and what steps they can take to pause surgery safely.

    (d) The anesthesiologist should take steps to simultaneously diagnose and treat MH, including hyperventilation, checking the ventilator circuit, checking the CO_2 absorbent, increasing flows of oxygen and air, checking the temperature probe, and drawing an arterial blood gas (ABG) to evaluate for combined metabolic and respiratory acidosis.

5. Phase 4: Initiation of malignant hyperthermia resuscitation protocol

    (a) Initial ABG will demonstrate combined metabolic and respiratory acidosis.

    (b) The patient will become increasingly hypercarbic, hyperthermia, tachycardic, and hypotensive.

    (c) The anesthesiologist should clearly communicate to the room (surgeon and nurse) that the patient is having a MH crisis. They should convey that this is an emergency and the patient will need to start resuscitation immediately, and it will require time and resources.

    (d) The anesthesiologist should ask the surgeon to abort surgery if possible. The surgeon should take steps to safely abort surgery and close the patient as fast as possible.

    (e) The anesthesiologist should activate the hospital MH protocol.

- Call for the MH cart.
- Call for the crash cart and defibrillator.
- Call an anesthesia STAT to enlist anesthesia technicians and additional personnel to help with resuscitation.
- Discontinue volatile anesthetic and convert to a total intravenous anesthetic (TIVA).
- Administer dantrolene 2.5 mg/kg IV, titrated up to 10 mg/kg IV pending symptom resolution.
- The anesthesia techs can assist with this: place charcoal filters in line with the ventilator circuit to prevent further administration of residual volatile anesthetic in the ventilation system. May hand bag with a Mapleson or Ambu-Bag to avoid this until a new ventilator or new parts (absorbent, circuit, etc.) can be replaced in the current ventilator.
- Ventilate with 100% FiO_2.
- Consider calling the Malignant Hyperthermia of the United States (MHAUS) hotline for additional guidance with the resuscitation.

- Treat presumed hyperkalemia: insulin 10 units IV, 1 ampule of dextrose 50%, albuterol, hyperventilation, calcium chloride 1000 mg, furosemide 10–20 mg IV, sodium bicarbonate 50 mEq.
- Place an arterial line and check serial ABGs to trend the resolution of metabolic and respiratory acidosis.
- Fluid resuscitate to prevent myoglobinuria. Starting fluid boluses include crystalloid 20–40 cc/kg IV titrated to hemodynamics and urine output. Goal urine output should be at least 0.5 cc/kg/h.
- Administer inotropes and pressors titrated to hemodynamic instability.
- Ask the nurse or surgeon to place a Foley catheter to monitor urine output.
- Cool patient to normothermia.
  - Since the abdomen is already open, the anesthesiologist may ask the surgeon to apply cold irrigation fluid to the abdomen to cool the patient.
- Establish large-bore intravenous access for large-volume resuscitation. The anesthesiologist may ask the surgeon to assist with placement of central line access, or the surgeon may offer, as the anesthesiologist will be occupied administering medications.
- Send labs including ABG, complete blood count, coagulation panel, basic metabolic panel, lactate, creatine kinase, and myoglobin.

(f) Note: There are many critical steps to be done. The anesthesiologist will be leading the resuscitation but should assign clear roles to all team members including the surgeons about how they can help. The resuscitation will be more efficient if each team member has specific tasks.

6. Phase 5: (Optional) Cardiac arrest
   (a) If the team does not enact the above interventions in a timely fashion, the patient will go into cardiac arrest. The simulation instructor can decide what arrhythmia and what the precise etiology is. An example may be ventricular tachycardia without a pulse secondary to hyperkalemia.
   (b) The team should follow Advanced Cardiac Life Support (ACLS) algorithms.

7. Phase 6: Disposition
   (a) If the above steps are performed appropriately, the patient will stabilize.
   (b) The team should discuss disposition planning, which should include remaining intubated and admitting the patient to the intensive care unit (ICU).
   (c) The team should acknowledge that the patient may continue to require dantrolene, volume resuscitation, inotropes and pressors, and serial labs to treat electrolyte disturbances.

Anesthesiology Scoring Rubric

Topic: Malignant hyperthermia			
Participants:			
Evaluators:			
Score:			
Tasks		Completed	Not completed
Initial development of hypercarbia and hyperthermia			
Evaluation and communication	Notify surgeons of hypercarbia and hyperthermia.		
	Notify surgeons of suspicion of malignant hyperthermia (MH) developing.		
	Ask surgeons to pause surgery if possible while evaluating for MH.		
Management	(If succinylcholine was used) Identify masseter muscle spasm and limited mouth opening.		
	(If masseter muscle spasm occurs) Discuss the difficulty of intubation and the potential for escalation to video laryngoscope or fiberoptic bronchoscope.		
	Recognize hypercarbia.		
	Increase minute ventilation by increasing respiratory rate and/or tidal volume.		
	Recognize hyperthermia.		
	Double-check ventilator equipment (settings, circuit, absorbent) and monitors to verify hypercarbia and hyperthermia.		
	Check the peripheral nerve stimulator to rule out inadequate muscle relaxation.		
	Recognize muscle rigidity as a symptom of MH.		
	Draw an initial arterial blood gas (ABG) to check for combined metabolic and respiratory acidosis.		

(continued)

Topic: Malignant hyperthermia			
Establishing diagnosis of malignant hyperthermia			
Evaluation and communication	Notify surgeons of the presence of a MH crisis and the need for resuscitation.		
	Adequately convey the severity and urgency of the situation to all staff.		
	Notify surgeons of worsening hemodynamic instability.		
	Notify surgeons of worsening hypercarbia and tachycardia.		
Management	Recognize the presence of combined metabolic and respiratory acidosis in the initial ABG.		
	Identify hemodynamic instability: Tachycardia and hypotension.		
Malignant hyperthermia resuscitation			
Evaluation and communication	Ask the surgeon to abort surgery as soon as possible.		
	Notify the operating room team of the need to initiate the MH protocol.		
	Call for the MH cart.		
	Call for the crash cart and defibrillator.		
	Call an anesthesia STAT to get additional personnel.		
	Clearly assign roles to all staff including surgeons, nurses, technicians, and other anesthesiologists.		
	May call the malignant hyperthermia of the United States (MHAUS) hotline.		
	Ask the surgeon/nurse to place a Foley catheter.		
	May ask the surgeon to help place additional lines such as a central line, arterial line, or peripheral IVs.		
	May ask the surgeon to irrigate the abdomen with a cold solution to help cool the patient.		
	May ask the surgeon to help reconstitute dantrolene vials.		

(continued)

Topic: Malignant hyperthermia			
Management	Administer dantrolene in appropriate doses, titrating appropriately to effect.		
	Discontinue volatile anesthetic.		
	Convert to total intravenous anesthetic (TIVA).		
	Ventilate with 100% FiO$_2$.		
	Any: Place charcoal filters; hand bag with a Mapleson or Ambu-Bag; change out parts of the current ventilator (absorbent, circuit, etc.); use the new ventilator.		
	Treat presumed hyperkalemia appropriately: Insulin, dextrose, hyperventilation, calcium chloride, furosemide, and sodium bicarbonate.		
	Place an arterial line.		
	Place a central line and large-bore peripheral IVs.		
	Check serial ABGs.		
	Evaluate acid-base status in labs to guide resuscitation.		
	Fluid resuscitates at adequate volumes.		
	Trend urine output with a clearly defined target.		
	Administer inotropes and vasopressors titrated to hemodynamics.		
	Send labs including ABG, CBC, coagulation panel, BMP, lactate, CK, and myoglobin.		
(Optional) Cardiac arrest			
Evaluation and communication	Notify the team that the patient is in cardiac arrest.		
	Notify the team that ACLS needs to be started.		
	Assign someone to do chest compressions.		
	Call out clear instructions for defibrillator settings.		

(continued)

Topic: Malignant hyperthermia			
Management	Correctly identify arrhythmia (e.g., ventricular tachycardia without a **pulse**).		
	Initiate ACLS in a timely fashion.		
	Start chest compressions in a timely fashion.		
	Appropriately defibrillate the patient in a timely fashion (e.g., unsynchronized cardioversion at 200 J).		
Disposition			
Evaluation and communication	Discuss with the surgeon the recommendation to remain intubated and be admitted to the ICU post-op.		
	Communicate to the surgeon that the patient will likely continue to need dantrolene doses and supportive care (e.g., fluids, pressors, inotropes).		

Postoperative Neck Hematoma

7

Scott Lewis and Claire Sampankanpanich Soria

7.1 Level of Training

- Anesthesiology resident
- General surgery resident

7.2 Learning Objectives

1. Review differential diagnoses for respiratory distress immediately post-extubation.
2. Review differential diagnoses for respiratory distress in the post-anesthesia care unit (PACU).
3. Review causes of airway compromise post-thyroidectomy.
4. Discuss management of emergent, difficult airway in the PACU.

7.3 Simulator Environment

1. Location: post-anesthesia care unit of a tertiary care center.
2. Manikin setup:
   (a) Age: adult.
   (b) Lines: 1 × 18 Gauge peripheral intravenous (PIV) line.
   (c) Monitors: non-invasive blood pressure (NIBP) cuff, 5-lead electrocardiogram (EKG), and pulse oximeter.
3. Medications available:
   (a) Fluids: normal saline, lactated ringers, and 5% albumin.

S. Lewis (✉) · C. S. Soria
University of California, San Diego, San Diego, CA, USA
e-mail: sjlewis@health.ucsd.edu; cssoria@health.ucsd.edu

© The Author(s), under exclusive license to Springer Nature Switzerland AG 2024
C. S. Soria, P. Yao (eds.), *Anesthesiology Simulation*,
https://doi.org/10.1007/978-3-031-80228-7_7

    (b) Blood products: none.

    (c) Sedatives/hypnotics: propofol, etomidate, and ketamine.

    (d) Paralytics: succinylcholine and rocuronium.

    (e) Cardiac agents: epinephrine, phenylephrine, ephedrine, atropine, glycopyrrolate, esmolol, labetalol, nicardipine, and dopamine.

    (f) Narcotics: midazolam, fentanyl, and hydromorphone.

4. Equipment available:

    (a) Airway equipment: Code bag (including mask, Mapleson, laryngoscope, and cuffed endotracheal tubes (ETTs) of various sizes, stylet, oral airway, nasal trumpet, laryngeal mask airway [LMA], bougie). Video laryngoscopes such as GlideScope or C-MAC and fiberoptic bronchoscope are available upon request, but there will be delay.

    (b) Monitors (none on patient initially but will be available upon request): NIBP cuff, 5-lead electrocardiogram (EKG), pulse oximeter, and end-tidal carbon dioxide ($ETCO_2$).

    (c) Lines (available upon request): arterial line kit and transducer, central line kit, and PIV kits.

    (d) Crash cart with defibrillator.

7.4   Actors

1. PACU nurse
2. Anesthesiologist
3. Surgeon

7.5   Case Narrative

1. Background:

    (a) At the start of the scenario, the surgeon is not initially involved. They should be in a separate room at the start of the scenario, unable to hear the initial Anesthesia STAT page to the anesthesiologist.

    (b) The surgeon should not be able to watch or hear what is happening in the simulation room. They will not enter the room until explicitly called for by the anesthesiologist.

    (c) The surgeon and anesthesiologist are on call at a tertiary care center.

    (d) The anesthesiologist receives an Anesthesia STAT page to their Code Blue pager that reads: "Anesthesia STAT, PACU Bay."

2. Phase 1: Initial assessment

    (a) Upon arrival, the anesthesiologist should perform a focused history and physical exam.

       • They will encounter a 65-year-old woman, obese, who is sitting upright in her gurney, struggling to breathe on simple face mask at 10 L/min O_2.

- There is audible inspiratory stridor and increased work of breathing, including use of accessory muscles of respiration, tracheal tugging, and intercostal retraction.
- There is gauze taped over the anterior neck that is soaked through with bright red blood.
- Per report, the patient's surgery did not have any complications. Regarding the patient's airway status, the patient was easy to bag mask ventilate and to intubate. They were extubated smoothly in the operating room at the end of the case.
- Other past medical history is notable for obstructive sleep apnea, obesity, hypertension, and goiter.
- The patient was sleeping upon arrival to the PACU, but after 1 h, woke up feeling nauseous and dry heaving. Within about 30 min, she became less talkative, had more bleeding from her surgical incision site, started to desaturate, and developed worsening respiratory distress.

(b) The anesthesiologist should ensure all monitors are on the patient.
   - Initial vital signs include BP 160s/80s, HR 110s, SpO_2 88%.

(c) The anesthesiologist should recognize that the patient has a rapidly expanding hematoma that will likely require surgical drainage and control of hemostasis.

(d) The anesthesiologist should call for the surgeon to bedside STAT.

(e) The anesthesiologist should notify the charge nurse/front desk of a possible level 1 takeback for neck hematoma evacuation.

(f) The anesthesiologist should call for a crash cart, anesthesia cart, and/or code bag to be brought to the PACU in case of need for emergent intubation in the PACU.

(g) The anesthesiologist should provide supplemental oxygen via Mapleson or Ambu Bag to provide 100% FiO_2 and potentially positive pressure ventilation.

(h) The anesthesiologist should prepare airway equipment and medications for possible emergent intubation. They may call for advanced airway equipment in anticipation of a difficult intubation, including a video laryngoscope, fiberoptic bronchoscope, and cricothyroidotomy kit.

3. Phase 2: Assessment of hematoma
   (a) The surgeon will arrive at bedside in a timely fashion.
   (b) The anesthesiologist should provide a concise report to the surgeon.
   (c) The surgeon and anesthesiologist should examine the neck and discuss how, where, and when to address the expanding hematoma and respiratory distress. Considerations will include:
      - Where is the safest place for surgical exploration of the neck hematoma?
         - The surgeon will likely prefer the operating room. If so, the team should mobilize the operating room nursing staff, surgery technicians, and anesthesia technicians to prepare for the operating room for emergency surgery.
      - Is the patient stable enough to transport quickly from the PACU to the OR?

- What is the safest way to intubate the patient? Options include asleep versus awake; direct laryngoscopy, video laryngoscopy, and fiberoptic bronchoscopy.
- What is the severity of tracheal deviation and mass compression due to the evolving hematoma? Should the surgical sutures be removed prior to intubation, to relieve the compression and improve chances of successful intubation?

4. Phase 3: Intubation
   (a) Prior to intubation, the surgeon should call for a cricothyroidotomy tray, prep the neck, and scrub, in case they need to perform an emergency cricothyroidotomy.
   (b) If the surgeon does not do this already, the anesthesiologist should ask the surgeon to prepare for an emergency surgical airway in case of loss of control of the airway.
   (c) The anesthesiologist may ask the surgeon to release the surgical sutures prior to induction and intubation.
   (d) Regardless of how and where the team decides to intubate, the patient will decompensate, become apneic, and desaturate.
   (e) The anesthesiologist will attempt to intubate. Regardless of whether they choose direct laryngoscopy, video laryngoscopy, or fiberoptic bronchoscopy, the anesthesiologist will have a grade 4 view and be unable to intubate due to mass compression and tracheal deviation. They will be unable to bag mask ventilate the patient.
   (f) The patient will continue to desaturate and will become hypotensive and bradycardic.
   (g) The anesthesiologist should notify the surgeon and ask them to release the surgical sutures.
   (h) The anesthesiologist should communicate clearly and frequently with the surgeon about airway status and whether the surgeon should proceed with an emergency cricothyroidotomy.
   (i) After the surgeon releases the surgical sutures, the anesthesiologist will note that bag mask ventilation is improving. The anesthesiologist will obtain a grade 2 view and be able to successfully intubate.

5. Phase 4: Surgical exploration
   (a) With the airway secured and adequate ventilation and oxygenation now secured, the surgeon can proceed with neck exploration and hemostasis.
   (b) The surgeon will encounter a venous bleed which they will be able to repair.
   (c) The surgeons and anesthesiologists should recap the events and discuss whether the patient is safe to extubate in the operating room.

(d) They will likely decide to keep the patient intubated and transport to the surgical intensive care unit (SICU) postoperatively for close observation.

7.6 Anesthesiology Scoring Rubric

Topic: PACU neck hematoma			
Participants:			
Evaluators:			
Score:			
Tasks		Completed	Not completed
Phase 1: Initial assessment			
Communication	Call for the surgeon to bedside STAT.		
	Notify the charge nurse/front desk of possible level 1 takeback for surgical exploration of the neck.		
	Call for a crash cart, anesthesia cart, and/or code bag.		
	Anticipate difficult intubation.		
Medical management	Perform a focused history and physical exam.		
	Ensure all monitors are on the patient.		
	Recognize that the patient has a rapidly expanding hematoma that needs surgical attention immediately.		
	Prepare equipment and medications for possible emergent intubation.		
	May call for advanced airway equipment in anticipation of a difficult intubation, including a video laryngoscope, fiberoptic bronchoscope, and cricothyroidotomy kit.		
	Provide supplemental oxygen via full face mask and Mapleson or Ambu Bag.		
Phase 2: Assessment of hematoma			
Communication	Provide a concise report to the surgeon.		
	Examine the neck with the surgeon.		
	Discuss with the surgeon how, when, and where to do the neck exploration.		
	Discuss with the surgeon how, when, and where to potentially intubate the patient.		
Phase 3: Intubation			
Communication	Ask the surgeons to prep the neck, scrub, and have a cricothyroidotomy tray ready to go in case a surgical airway is needed emergently.		
	May ask the surgeon to release the surgical sutures prior to induction and intubation.		
	Notify the surgeon that they have a grade 4 view secondary to severe mass compression.		
	Notify the surgeon that they are unable to bag mask ventilate.		
	Ask the surgeon to release the surgical sutures.		
	Communicate clearly and frequently with the surgeon about airway status and whether the surgeon should proceed with an emergency cricothyroidotomy.		

(continued)

Topic: PACU neck hematoma			
Medical management	Perform initial intubation attempt (any method is acceptable).		
	Attempt bag mask ventilation.		
	After suture release, re-attempt intubation.		
Phase 4: Surgical exploration			
Communication	Debrief with surgeon about recent events and current airway and hemodynamic status.		
	Discuss with the surgeon disposition planning and whether it is safe to extubate in the operating room.		
Medical management	Keep the patient intubated and transport to the intensive care unit for close observation.		

Power Outage

8

Claire Sampankanpanich Soria

8.1 Level of Training

- Anesthesiology resident
- General surgery resident

8.2 Learning Objectives

1. Review anticipated hemodynamic changes of insufflation during laparoscopic surgery.
2. Discuss equipment failures that would be affected by a power outage.
3. Highlight alternative methods for maintaining ventilation and depth of anesthesia during a power outage.
4. Discuss potential surgical complications of losing video visualization and insufflation pressures during laparoscopic surgery.
5. Review strategies performing surgery during a power outage.

8.3 Simulator Environment

1. Location: main operating room of an outpatient surgical center.
2. Manikin setup:
   (a) Age: adult.
   (b) Lines: 1 × 18 gauge (G) peripheral intravenous (PIV) in the hand.
   (c) Monitors: non-invasive blood pressure (NIBP) cuff, 5-lead electrocardiogram (EKG), pulse oximeter, and temperature probe.

C. S. Soria (✉)
University of California, San Diego, San Diego, CA, USA
e-mail: cssoria@health.ucsd.edu

© The Author(s), under exclusive license to Springer Nature Switzerland AG 2024
C. S. Soria, P. Yao (eds.), *Anesthesiology Simulation*,
https://doi.org/10.1007/978-3-031-80228-7_8

3. Medications available:
   (a) Fluids: normal saline, lactated ringers, and 5% albumin.
   (b) Sedatives/hypnotics: propofol, etomidate, and inhaled anesthetics.
   (c) Paralytics: succinylcholine and rocuronium.
   (d) Cardiac agents: epinephrine, phenylephrine, ephedrine, vasopressin, atropine, glycopyrrolate, esmolol, labetalol, nicardipine, and dopamine.
   (e) Narcotics: midazolam, fentanyl, and hydromorphone.
4. Equipment available:
   (a) Airway equipment: anesthesia ventilator (including circuit, mask, suction), laryngoscope and cuffed endotracheal tubes (ETTs) of various sizes, stylet, oropharyngeal airway, nasopharyngeal airway, laryngeal mask airway (LMA), and bougie. Video laryngoscope and fiberoptic bronchoscope are available if specifically requested by the learner.
   (b) Monitors: pulse oximeter, blood pressure cuff, 5-lead EKG, and $ETCO_2$ monitor.
   (c) Lines: arterial line kit, central line kit, including triple lumen and Cordis, and PIV kits available upon request.
   (d) Crash cart with defibrillator is outside in the hallway and available upon request.

8.4   Actors

1. Surgeon
2. Anesthesiologist
3. Circulator nurse
4. Surgical scrub technician
5. Anesthesia technician

8.5   Case Narrative

1. Scenario background given to participants:
   (a) You are the anesthesia and surgical team working at an outpatient surgical center.
   (b) The patient is a 60-year-old man, 6′, 80 kg, BMI 23.9, with mild gastroesophageal reflux disease (GERD) and well-controlled hypertension (HTN) who is undergoing laparoscopic umbilical hernia repair.
   (c) Past medical history: mild GERD and well-controlled HTN.
   (d) Medications: labetalol and omeprazole.
   (e) Allergies: none.
   (f) Past surgical history: tonsillectomy at age 5 years old.
   (g) Labs: none.
2. Phase 1: Induction

(a) The anesthesia and surgery teams will perform a timeout prior to induction, confirming equipment, allergies, fire risk, correct patient, and site.

(b) The anesthesiologist will perform a routine induction and intubation. This will be uneventful. The patient will be easy to intubate and will remain hemodynamically stable through induction.

3. Phase 2: Insufflation

(a) The surgeons will proceed with starting the surgery, including prepping the patient, positioning, inserting trocars, and beginning insufflation.

(b) The patient will become slightly bradycardic to a heart rate (HR) of low 50s bpm but maintain mean arterial pressure (MAP) in the 60s mmHg.

(c) The surgeon should notify the anesthesiologist that they have insufflated and may inquire whether the patient is tolerating insufflation well.

(d) The anesthesiologist may elect to treat the bradycardia with a medication like glycopyrrolate or ephedrine, a fluid bolus, or may choose to wait and observe. The anesthesiologist should be clear about the patient status and that it is fine for the surgeon to proceed.

4. Phase 3: Power outage

(a) As the surgeons continue working, there will suddenly be a power outage in the entire operating room.

(b) All equipment and lights will turn off. This will include room lights, overhead lights, ventilator, suction, monitors, computers, phones, cameras, surgical towers, and electrocautery. Gas lines will still be intact, including oxygen, air, and nitrous oxide.

(c) The insufflation will drop to a pressure of zero and the abdomen will desufflate while the instruments and trocars are still in the abdomen without video camera visualization.

(d) The anesthesiologist and surgeon should communicate about which of their equipment is not working and the current patient status from their perspective as surgeon and anesthesiologist.

(e) The team should call for an anesthesia STAT to summon more help. This will need to be done by sending a runner out of the operating room, as the phone and intercom system will be down.

(f) The team should look for portable light sources so they can see, especially in the surgical field. This may include emergency flashlights, pen lights, and cellular phone lights.

5. Phase 4: Management

(a) Anesthesiologist tasks:

- The anesthesiologist should ensure adequate oxygenation and ventilation by switching the patient from the ventilator to manual bagging via the in situ ETT. This can be achieved by using a Mapleson or Ambu Bag connected to the auxiliary oxygen port on the ventilator or a portable oxygen tank.

- The anesthesiologist should call for a portable monitor to place on the patient to continue to monitor vital signs. This may include a full transport monitor that is capable of electrocardiogram (EKG), blood pressure

(BP), and pulse oximetry (SpO_2), but the transport monitor may or may not have end-tidal carbon dioxide ($ETCO_2$) capabilities. If a full transport monitor is unavailable, the anesthesiologist may use a pulse oximeter monitor, which would provide pulse oximetry and heart rate but not rhythm.

- The anesthesiologist should maintain the patient under general anesthesia to maintain analgesia, hypnosis, and lack of movement. They will need to do this using a total intravenous anesthetic (TIVA) because their ventilator will not power on and they will be unable to deliver inhaled anesthetics such as nitrous oxide or volatile anesthetic. The learner will likely opt to administer a propofol infusion or boluses of propofol, ketamine, and/or dexmedetomidine. If the learner has infusion pumps in the room, they will have enough battery power in them to last for a few hours until the power outage resolves.
- The anesthesiologist may be concerned about intraoperative awareness, especially if there is a delay in initiating the TIVA. The anesthesiologist may choose to administer midazolam and ketamine to prevent this.
- The anesthesiologist should communicate with the surgeon about patient hemodynamic stability. This will help guide the surgeon to know if the patient is having a surgical complication such as bleeding or trauma from the instruments and loss of insufflation that needs to be surgically repaired.
- While the patient is off monitors, the anesthesiologist may palpate for a carotid pulse to check blood pressure qualitatively. The anesthesiologist may also use a light source to check coloration for cyanosis.

(b) Surgeon tasks:
- The surgeon will need to determine whether they are in a stage of surgery where they can abort and quickly close the patient's current incisions.
- They will be unable to see anything laparoscopically as their surgical monitor and towers will have lost all power and have no battery reserve option.
- If the surgeon decides they are unable to remove the trocars and instruments and close, they may decide to open the patient and operate under flashlights to finish the surgery in the abdomen and close.
- If the surgeon is at a point where it is ok to remove the trocars and instruments and close, they may do so.
- Depending on what surgical steps have been done so far in the scenario, the simulation instructor may decide to have a small degree of bleeding in the scenario for the surgeons to address.
- The surgeon should communicate with the anesthesiologist about the timeframe for when they can close the patient or if they need more time to do things like open the patient and repair any potential damage.

6. Phase 5: Resolution
   (a) The surgeons will be able to quickly abort the surgery and close the patient.

(b) The anesthesiologist will be able to emerge the patient from general anesthesia and safely extubate without complication.

8.6   Anesthesiology Scoring Rubric

Topic: Power outage		Completed	Not completed
Participants:			
Evaluators:			
Score:			
Tasks		Completed	Not completed
Insufflation pre-power outage			
Medical management	Recognize bradycardia developing after insufflation of the abdomen and check blood pressure for associated hypotension.		
	Treat the bradycardia with pressors and/or fluid bolus.		
Communication	Appropriately reassure surgeons that the bradycardia is likely a normal physiologic response to peritoneal stretching from insufflation of the abdomen and that it is safe to proceed.		
Post-power outage			
Medical management	Check all equipment and monitors to identify what is or is not working.		
	Re-establish oxygenation and ventilation in a timely fashion using Mapleson or Ambu Bag with alternate oxygen source (tank or auxiliary port on ventilator).		
	Call for anesthesia STAT, anesthesia technician, and additional personnel.		
	Initiate total intravenous anesthetic in a timely fashion.		
	Administer appropriate medications to ensure lack of awareness, lack of pain, and lack of patient movement.		
	Place patient on alternative monitors such as transport monitor or portable pulse oximeter.		
	While the patient is off monitors, palpate carotid pulse to assess blood pressure and perfusion.		
	Locate alternative light source like flashlight or cell phone light.		
	While the patient is off monitors, use light source to observe the patient's coloration and check for cyanosis indicative of inadequate oxygenation and ventilation.		
	At the end of surgery, perform awake extubation in the operating room.		

(continued)

Topic: Power outage			
Communication	Update surgeons regularly on the status of anesthesia equipment and depth of anesthesia.		
	Update surgeons regularly on the patient's hemodynamic stability or changes in vital signs.		
	Ask surgeons about the timeframe for finishing surgery or if any surgical complications have occurred that would delay closure.		

Venous Air Embolism

9

Claire Sampankanpanich Soria

9.1 Level of Training

– Anesthesiology resident
– General surgery resident

9.2 Learning Objectives

1. Discuss the signs and symptoms of a venous air embolism (VAE)
2. Review the pathophysiology of a VAE
3. Review the treatment and prevention of a VAE

9.3 Simulator Environment

1. Operating room of an outpatient surgical center:
2. Manikin setup:
   (a) Age: adult.
   (b) Lines: 1 × 18-gauge (G) peripheral intravenous (PIV) in the hand.
   (c) Monitors: non-invasive blood pressure (NIBP) cuff, 5-lead electrocardiogram (EKG), pulse oximeter, and temperature probe.
3. Medications available:
   (a) Fluids: normal saline, lactated Ringer's solution, and 5% albumin.
   (b) Blood products: 2 units of packed red blood cells (PRBCs).
   (c) Sedatives/hypnotics: propofol, etomidate, ketamine, and inhaled anesthetics.
   (d) Paralytics: succinylcholine and rocuronium.

C. S. Soria (✉)
University of California, San Diego, San Diego, CA, USA
e-mail: cssoria@health.ucsd.edu

© The Author(s), under exclusive license to Springer Nature Switzerland AG 2024
C. S. Soria, P. Yao (eds.), *Anesthesiology Simulation*,
https://doi.org/10.1007/978-3-031-80228-7_9

  (e) Cardiac agents: epinephrine, phenylephrine, ephedrine, vasopressin, atropine, glycopyrrolate, esmolol, labetalol, nicardipine, and dopamine.

  (f) Narcotics: midazolam, fentanyl, and hydromorphone.

4. Equipment available:

  (a) Airway equipment: anesthesia ventilator (including circuit, mask, and suction), laryngoscopes, and cuffed endotracheal tubes (ETTs) of various sizes, stylet, oropharyngeal airway, nasopharyngeal airway, laryngeal mask airway (LMA), and bougie. Video laryngoscope and fiberoptic bronchoscope are available if specifically requested by the learner.

  (b) Monitors: pulse oximeter, blood pressure cuff, 5-lead EKG, and end-tidal carbon dioxide ($ETCO_2$) monitor. Additional monitors such as arterial line transducer, central venous pressure (CVP) transducer, and trans-esophageal echocardiogram (TEE) are available if specifically requested by the learner.

  (c) Lines: arterial line kit, central line kit, including triple lumen, Cordis, and air retrieval catheter, and PIV kits are available upon request.

  (d) A crash cart with a defibrillator is outside the room and available upon request.

9.4 Actors

1. Surgeon
2. Anesthesiologist
3. Circulator nurse
4. Surgical scrub technician
5. Anesthesia technician

9.5 Case Narrative

1. Scenario background given to participants

  (a) You are the anesthesia and surgical team working at an outpatient surgical center.

  (b) The patient is a 25-year-old woman, with a height of 5′5″, a weight of 90 kg, and a body mass index (BMI) of 33.3. She has a history of obesity and childhood asthma and is undergoing laparoscopic cholecystectomy for symptomatic cholelithiasis.

  (c) Past medical history: obesity, asthma as a child, never hospitalized, never intubated, and has not required a rescue albuterol inhaler since she was a teenager.

  (d) Medications: none.

  (e) Allergies: none.

  (f) Past surgical history: laparoscopic appendectomy for acute appendicitis when she was 19 years old; laparoscopic ovarian cystectomy for dermoid cyst when she was 23 years old.

(g) Labs: hemoglobin 13.0, hematocrit 39.0, and platelets 200K.
2. Phase 1: Induction
   (a) The anesthesia and surgery teams will perform a timeout prior to induction, confirming equipment, allergies, fire risk, and correct patient and site.
   (b) The anesthesiologist will perform a routine induction and intubation. This will be uneventful. The patient will be easy to intubate and will remain hemodynamically stable through induction.
3. Phase 2: Insertion of trocars
   (a) The surgeons will insert the trocars. They will note that the patient has extensive scar tissue. Eventually, the surgeon will begin insufflation of the abdomen.
   (b) Unknowingly, the surgeon will have inserted the insufflation needle into a vein.
4. Phase 3: Drop in end-tidal carbon dioxide (ETCO$_2$)
   (a) The patient will be hemodynamically stable up until this point in the case.
   (b) Suddenly, the ETCO$_2$ will change: It may initially increase from absorption of ETCO$_2$ but will then drop precipitously without any previous change in ventilator settings, as an air lock occurs and there is decreased perfusion to the pulmonary circulation.
   (c) The capnogram waveform will have normal tracing qualitatively.
   (d) Simultaneously, the patient will become acutely tachycardic and hypotensive. Initially, the patient will be in sinus tachycardia (e.g., heart rate [HR] 140s and systolic blood pressure [SBP] 70s).
5. Phase 4: Initial communication about a problem
   (a) The anesthesiologist should recognize the acute drop in ETCO$_2$, hypotension, and tachycardia.
   (b) The anesthesiologist should notify the surgeon of the hemodynamic instability and drop in ETCO$_2$.
   (c) The anesthesiologist should ask the surgeon to check for a surgical etiology.
   (d) The anesthesiologist should simultaneously diagnose and treat:
       • Check the ventilator settings, circuit, and ETT, auscultate breath sounds, and manually bag the patient to assess compliance.
       • Recycle the blood pressure cuff.
       • May palpate for a pulse manually.
       • Administer a fluid bolus.
       • Administer pressors and/or inotropes.
       • Go to 100% fraction of inspired oxygen (FiO$_2$).
   (e) The anesthesiologist should have a high suspicion for VAE, hemorrhage, or tension pneumothorax but may consider other differential diagnoses such as anaphylaxis and medication error.
6. Phase 5: Initial evaluation
   (a) The surgeon should survey their surgical field to check for sources of bleeding and confirm the appropriate positioning of their needles.

(b) The surgeon will not find any evidence of major bleeding in the abdomen but will find that the insufflation needle appears to have punctured a blood vessel.

(c) The anesthesiologist should ask the surgeon to desufflate the abdomen at this time, to avoid further insufflation of the carbon dioxide embolus into the vascular system.

(d) The patient's hemodynamics will transiently improve with fluids and pressors.

(e) If the team does not desufflate the abdomen, then ventilation and oxygenation will continue to worsen.

(f) The patient will desaturate, and the $ETCO_2$ will continue to drop as cardiac output declines.

7. Phase 6: Management of venous air embolism
   (a) The surgeon should desufflate the abdomen.
   (b) The anesthesiologist should provide supportive care, including:
   - Administering a fluid bolus.
   - Providing inotropic or pressor support as needed.
   - Ensuring adequate oxygenation and ventilation.
   (c) The anesthesiologist may place an arterial line to draw arterial blood gases (ABGs) and evaluate for hypoxemia and respiratory acidosis.
   - Initial ABG will show respiratory acidosis and hypoxemia: 7.25/70/40/24.
   (d) The anesthesiologist may call for and insert a TEE probe to evaluate for right heart strain and visualize the presence of air in the heart.
   - TEE will show dilated right ventricle, tricuspid regurgitation, D-shaped right ventricle, and bowing of interventricular septum into the left ventricle. Also, large amount of air are present in all four ventricles, more on the right side than the left side.
   (e) The anesthesiologist may call to reposition the patient into the left lateral decubitus position. This may prevent further air from going into the pulmonary circulation.
   (f) The anesthesiologist may attempt to place an air retrieval catheter in the internal jugular vein to try to remove the VAE.
   - They will aspirate over 20 cc of air from the air retrieval catheter.

8. Phase 7: (Optional) Cardiac arrest
   (a) If the team does not enact the above interventions in a timely fashion, the patient will go into cardiac arrest. The simulation instructor can decide what arrhythmia is and what the precise etiology is. An example may be ventricular tachycardia without a pulse secondary to hyperkalemia.
   (b) The team should follow advanced cardiac life support (ACLS) algorithms.

9. Phase 8: Disposition
   (a) If the above steps are performed appropriately, the patient will stabilize.

(b) The team should discuss disposition planning, which will likely include remaining intubated and admitting the patient to the intensive care unit (ICU) for continued supportive care.

9.6   Anesthesiology Scoring Rubric

Topic: Venous air embolism			
Participants:			
Evaluators:			
Score:			
Tasks		Completed	Not completed
Development of problems with ventilation and hemodynamic instability			
Evaluation and communication	Notify the surgeon about new-onset hemodynamic instability and problems with ventilation		
	Ask the surgeon to survey their surgical field for possible etiology		
Management	Recognize the initial drop in $ETCO_2$		
	Recognize the presence of hypotension and tachycardia		
	Double-check ventilator settings, circuit, and ETT, auscultate breath sounds, and assess compliance on manual bagging		
	Double-check vitals such as re-cycling the blood pressure cuff, may palpate for pulse manually		
	Administer a fluid bolus		
	Administer pressors and/or inotropes		
	Increase FiO_2 to 100%		
	Develop differential diagnosis (e.g., VAE, hemorrhage, tension pneumothorax, and anaphylaxis)		
	Recognize that the insufflation needle in the blood vessel is the source of a VAE		
Management of venous air embolism			
Evaluation and communication	Ask the surgeon to desufflate the abdomen		
Management	Continue providing supportive care		
	May place an arterial line to draw ABGs and evaluate for hypoxemia and respiratory acidosis		
	May place a TEE probe to evaluate for right heart strain and visualize the presence of air in the heart		
	May reposition the patient into the left lateral decubitus position		
	May place an air retrieval catheter in the internal jugular vein and try to aspirate air		

(continued)

Topic: Venous air embolism			
(Optional) Cardiac arrest			
Evaluation and communication	Notify the team that the patient is in cardiac arrest		
	Notify the team that ACLS needs to be started		
	Assign someone to do chest compressions		
	Call out clear instructions for defibrillator settings		
Management	Correctly identify arrhythmia (e.g., ventricular tachycardia without a pulse)		
	Initiate ACLS in a timely fashion		
	Start chest compressions in a timely fashion		
	Appropriately defibrillate the patient in a timely fashion (e.g., unsynchronized cardioversion at 200 J)		
Disposition			
Evaluation and communication	Discuss with the surgeon the recommendation to remain intubated and admit to the ICU post-op.		
	Communicate to the surgeon that the patient may need continued supportive care such as inotropes and pressors		

Malfunctioning Tracheostomy

10

Scott Lewis and Claire Sampankanpanich Soria

10.1 Level of Training

- Anesthesiology resident
- General surgery resident

10.2 Learning Objectives

1. Review how to troubleshoot tracheostomies
2. Discuss navigating medical ethics concerns in acute emergencies
3. Review the advanced cardiac life support (ACLS) algorithm.

10.3 Simulator Environment

1. Location: inpatient floor in a tertiary care center.
2. Manikin setup:
   (a) Age: adult.
   (b) Lines: 1 × 20-gauge peripheral intravenous (PIV) line.
3. Medications available:
   (a) Fluids: normal saline and lactated Ringer's solution.
   (b) Blood products: none.
   (c) Sedatives/hypnotics: propofol and etomidate.
   (d) Paralytics: succinylcholine and rocuronium.
   (e) Cardiac agents: epinephrine, phenylephrine, ephedrine, and atropine.
4. Equipment available:

S. Lewis (✉) · C. S. Soria
University of California, San Diego, San Diego, CA, USA
e-mail: sjlewis@health.ucsd.edu; cssoria@health.ucsd.edu

C. S. Soria, P. Yao (eds.), *Anesthesiology Simulation*,
https://doi.org/10.1007/978-3-031-80228-7_10

(a) Airway equipment: code bag (including mask, Mapleson, laryngoscopes and cuffed endotracheal tubes [ETTs] of various sizes, stylet, oral airway, nasal trumpet, laryngeal mask airway [LMA], and bougie). Video laryngoscopes such as GlideScope or C-MAC and fiberoptic bronchoscope are available upon request, but there will be a delay.

(b) Monitors (none on patient initially but will be available upon request): non-invasive blood pressure (NIBP) cuff, five-lead electrocardiogram (EKG), pulse oximeter, and end-tidal carbon dioxide ($ETCO_2$).

(c) Lines (available upon request): arterial line kit and transducer, central line kit, and PIV kits.

(d) Crash cart with defibrillator.

10.4 Actors

1. Surgical team
2. Anesthesia team
3. Primary nurse
4. Rapid response nurse
5. Respiratory therapist

10.5 Case Narrative

1. Background:
   (a) At the start of the scenario, the surgeon is not initially involved. They should be in a separate room, unable to hear the initial code blue page to the anesthesiologist.
   (b) The surgeon should not be able to watch or hear what is happening in the simulation room. They will not enter the room until explicitly called for by the anesthesiologist.
   (c) The surgeon and anesthesiologist are on call at a tertiary care center.
   (d) The anesthesiologist receives an anesthesia STAT page to their code blue pager that reads: "Anesthesia STAT, Inpatient Floor, Trach not working, desaturation."
2. Phase 1: Initial survey
   (a) The anesthesiologist will be provided a "code bag" for the scenario, which contains basic airway equipment and medications typically found in a standard code bag.
   (b) The anesthesiologist should perform a focused history and physical examination and a quick survey of the scene.
      • They will observe that there is only the primary nurse, the on-call internal medicine intern, and a respiratory therapist at the bedside.
      • The patient appears to be bleeding from his neck, and the tracheostomy tube is hanging out of the stoma.

- The team is trying to calm the patient down. He appears to be confused and agitated and is trying to get out of bed.
- There are no monitors on the patient initially.
- There is an audible stridor coming from the patient, who appears uncomfortable and panicked.

(c) The anesthesiologist should identify the current code leader and ask for a status update and events leading up to the current situation.

(d) The anesthesiologist should determine whether the patient is in cardiac arrest or respiratory arrest and follow the ACLS algorithm appropriately.

(e) The anesthesiologist should physically position themselves at the head of the bed, as their primary focus is the airway.

(f) The anesthesiologist should instruct the nurse to place monitors on the patient: NIBP, EKG, and pulse oximetry (SpO_2).
  - Initial vital signs: heart rate (HR) 110 sinus rhythm, NIBP 150/90, and SpO_2 88% on room air.

(g) The anesthesiologist should evaluate the airway and determine how severe the patient's respiratory distress is:
  - The patient will be spontaneously breathing but with a loud, audible inspiratory stridor.
  - The patient will be using accessory muscles of respiration and display tracheal tugging and intercostal retractions.

(h) Upon request, the following history will be provided:
  - The patient is a 70-year-old man with a tracheostomy tube placed 2 years ago. He was admitted to the hospital 3 days ago from a nursing home for community-acquired pneumonia. Past medical history is notable for dementia and vocal cord paralysis secondary to complications from thyroidectomy for thyroid cancer. He never underwent radiation only chemotherapy and surgical resection, but he has been tracheostomy-dependent.
  - The patient has been delirious since being hospitalized. Earlier in the night shift, he was pulling at his PIV and his tracheostomy tube. When the nurse returned to his room to check on him, they found him bleeding from the neck. The team thinks he may have traumatized his tracheostomy site, resulting in the bleeding.

3. Phase 2: Airway management

(a) The anesthesiologist should provide supplemental oxygen to the patient. This can be a simple face mask, non-rebreather, but preferably a Mapleson that can deliver 100% fraction of inspired oxygen (FiO_2) with an appropriate seal and enable the provision of positive pressure. The anesthesiologist may consider placing a face mask over the tracheostomy stoma given there will be an air leak or may opt not to given the presence of bleeding from the stoma site.

(b) Early on in the resuscitation, the anesthesiologist should ask the team to page trauma surgery (who is in-house) and/or otolaryngology (though they are not typically in-house) for assistance in managing the stoma bleed.

    (c) The anesthesiologist should deduce based on the history that the patient is intubatable from the oropharynx or nasopharynx.

    (d) The anesthesiologist may consider the administration of heliox given the stridor. This will take time but can be provided in the scenario if requested.

    (e) The anesthesiologist should consider intubating the patient orally so there is a secure airway, until the bleeding at the stoma site can be repaired. If they choose to pursue intubation, the anesthesiologist should downsize their ETT in the setting of vocal cord paralysis.

    (f) The anesthesiologist should call for a video laryngoscope and a fiberoptic bronchoscope.

    (g) The anesthesiologist may ask someone to review the patient's electronic medical records for intubation history to determine whether the patient has a potentially difficult airway, aside from the stridor secondary to vocal cord paralysis.

    (h) Upon doing so, the team will learn that the patient has a "Do Not Intubate (DNI)" code status.

4. Phase 3: Code status and tracheostomy assessment

    (a) The surgeon will arrive at the bedside quickly.

    (b) The anesthesiologist should provide a concise report to the surgeon.

    (c) The surgeon should evaluate the stoma bleeding.
- They will note that it appears to be a venous bleed secondary to a laceration or tear, likely created by the patient scratching or pulling at his tracheostomy tube.

    (d) The team must decide how to address the DNI code status.
- The patient will be unable to consent for himself due to his delirium and dementia.
- The team may try to call a family member for consent, but will be unable to reach anyone.
- The team may bring up the idea of consulting a member of the ethics committee, but they will be unavailable in the middle of the night.
- The team should proceed with intubation and securement of the airway.

5. Phase 4: Intubation and repair of tracheostomy stoma bleed

    (a) The surgeon and anesthesiologist should discuss jointly how to secure the airway and how and where to repair the tracheal bleed.
- Considerations include:
  - Is the patient safe for transport?
  - How long can the patient maintain adequate oxygenation and ventilation given the severity of their stridor and increased work of breathing?
  - Is the patient anticipated to have difficult bag-mask ventilation and/or difficult intubation?
  - Where is the safest place to intubate the patient based on this information?
  - Where is the safest or most convenient place for the surgeon to evaluate and survey the stoma bleed?

- One possibility is to intubate orally with a downsized ETT at the bedside and then transport the patient to the operating room for repair of the tracheal bleed.

(b) Ultimately, the anesthesiologist will be able to successfully intubate the patient.

(c) The surgeon will be able to repair the laceration and venous bleed at the stoma site.

(d) The team should discuss when to replace the tracheostomy tube in the stoma site and remove the oral ETT. The scenario will end after this verbal discussion.

10.6   Anesthesiology Scoring Rubric

Topic: Code blue/DNI/Trach		Completed	Not completed
Participants:			
Evaluators:			
Score:			
Tasks		Completed	Not completed
Initial survey/arrival at the bedside			
Communication	Identify the code leader		
	Ask for a status update/recent events		
	Ask the nurse to place a full set of monitors (NIBP, EKG, and SpO$_2$)		
Medical management	Perform a focused history, physical examination, and survey of the scene		
	Position self at the head of the bed		
	Examine the airway and work of breathing		
Airway management			
Communication	Ask the nurse to page trauma surgery, maybe also ear, nose, and throat (ENT)		
	Discuss the possibility of intubating the patient orally		
	May ask the nurse/respiratory therapist to call for heliox		
	Check electronic medical record (EMR) for intubation history and confirm intubatable from oropharynx/nasopharynx		
	Call for video laryngoscope and/or fiberoptic bronchoscope		
Medical management	Provide supplemental oxygen to the face: Simple face mask, non-rebreather, and Mapleson		
	May provide supplemental oxygen at the tracheostomy stoma site		
	If moving to intubate, downsize ETT		

(continued)

Topic: Code blue/DNI/Trach			
Code status/tracheostomy assessment			
Communication	Provide a concise sign-out to the surgeon		
	Discuss with the surgeon how to proceed given DNI		
	May try to call a family member for consent		
	May discuss calling the ethics committee		
Medical management	Proceed with intubation and airway securement		
Intubation and repair of stoma bleed			
Communication	Discuss with the surgeon how and where to intubate		
	Discuss with the surgeon how and where to repair the stoma bleed		
	Discuss when to replace the tracheostomy tube after the stoma bleed repair		
Medical management	Intubate the patient in a timely fashion with a downsized ETT		

Difficult Airway in Obstetrics

11

Claire Sampankanpanich Soria

11.1 Level of Training

– Anesthesiology resident
– Obstetrics/gynecology resident

11.2 Learning Objectives

1. Review the anesthetic options for an emergency cesarean section
2. Discuss the anesthetic management of a difficult airway in obstetric anesthesia

11.3 Simulator Environment

1. Location: obstetrics operating room (OR) of a tertiary care center.
2. Manikin setup:
   (a) Age: adult.
   (b) Lines: 1 × 20-gauge peripheral intravenous (PIV) line.
3. Medications available:
   (a) Fluids: normal saline, lactated Ringer's solution, and albumin.
   (b) Blood products: 2 units of packed red blood cells (PRBCs).
   (c) Sedatives/hypnotics: propofol and etomidate.
   (d) Paralytics: succinylcholine and rocuronium.
   (e) Cardiac agents: epinephrine, phenylephrine, ephedrine, atropine, vasopressin, norepinephrine, and dopamine.
4. Equipment available:

C. S. Soria (✉)
University of California, San Diego, San Diego, CA, USA
e-mail: cssoria@health.ucsd.edu

(a) Airway equipment: face mask, Mapleson, laryngoscopes and cuffed endotracheal tubes (ETTs) of various sizes, stylet, oral airway, nasal trumpet, laryngeal mask airway (LMA), and bougie. Video laryngoscopes such as GlideScope or C-MAC and fiberoptic bronchoscope (FOB) are available upon request, but there will be a delay.

(b) Monitors (none on patient initially but will be available upon request): non-invasive blood pressure (NIBP) cuff, five-lead electrocardiogram (EKG), pulse oximeter, and end-tidal carbon dioxide ($ETCO_2$).

(c) Lines (available upon request): arterial line kit and transducer, central line kit, and PIV kits.

(d) Crash cart with defibrillator.

(e) Trans-esophageal echocardiogram (TEE) and trans-thoracic echocardiogram (TTE) are available upon request.

11.4 Actors

1. Obstetrics/gynecology team
2. Anesthesia team
3. Circulator nurse
4. Scrub technician
5. Anesthesia technician

11.5 Case Narrative

1. Background:
   (a) The obstetrician–gynecologist (OB/GYN) surgeon and anesthesiologist are on call at a tertiary care center.
   (b) The anesthesiologist receives a page that reads, "CODE PINK OR1."
      • Upon arrival in the OR, they will note that the patient is a 25-year-old woman, with a large body mass index (BMI; appears morbidly obese), who is hyperventilating and in significant pain from active labor. The patient has one 22 G PIV in the hand.
      • The OB/GYN team is in the process of moving the patient from the gurney to the OR table. The patient is not on monitors yet.
   (c) The OB/GYN surgeon will have additional information about the patient, provided to them on a sheet of paper for the scenario. The surgeon and anesthesiologist will need to speak with each other to share this information.
   (d) Background information is to be provided on a piece of paper to the OB/GYN surgeon only. This is not to be given to the anesthesiologist.
      • The patient has housing insecurity and has not had regular prenatal care.
      • This is her fourth pregnancy. She has had one prior cesarean section, one spontaneous abortion, and one successful vaginal birth after the cesarean section.

- The patient arrived in the emergency room 20 min ago and was found to be in active labor with a breech presentation. Fetal heart rate (FHR) was initially reassuring, but now the obstetrics nurse and obstetrician have had difficulty obtaining FHR tracing, and when they do, there is minimal activity.
- A crash section was called due to breech presentation and fetal distress.
- The obstetrician wants to proceed with an emergency cesarean section. They have determined there is no time for the anesthesiologist to attempt a neuraxial block. The obstetrician wants to proceed with general anesthesia.

2. Phase 1: Initial survey
   (a) The anesthesiologist should place the patient on full monitors, including pulse oximetry (SpO$_2$), NIBP, and 5-lead EKG.
   (b) Starting vital signs are as follows: systolic blood pressure (SBP) is in the 90s mmHg, SpO$_2$ is 98% on room air, and heart rate (HR) is in the 120s with sinus tachycardia.
   (c) The anesthesiologist should simultaneously assess and treat the patient/fetus.
   - The anesthesiologist should place the patient on supplemental oxygen such as via a simple face mask to improve oxygenation and perfusion to the uterus. The anesthesiologist may use the circuit mask in anticipation of needing pre-oxygenation for general anesthesia.
   - The anesthesiologist should administer a fluid bolus and pressor to support the patient's blood pressure and try to increase perfusion pressure to the uterus.
   (d) The anesthesiologist should seek additional information about the patient, including past medical history, history of present illness, current vascular access, resuscitation measures implemented so far, recent labs, and blood products available. They may try to obtain this information by interviewing the patient, reviewing the electronic medical record, and speaking with the OB/GYN surgeon.
   (e) The OB/GYN surgeon should provide the information they have to the anesthesiologist in a timely fashion.
   (f) The OB/GYN surgeon should clearly set expectations with the anesthesiologist about the timing of when they want to perform the cesarean section and what anesthetic management they want: In this case, it will be a true emergency cesarean section with no time for the anesthesiologist to attempt neuraxial blockade. It must be done under general anesthesia.

3. Phase 2: Induction
   (a) The anesthesiologist should pre-oxygenate the patient and prepare for anticipated challenging intubation, given the patient's morbid obesity, gravid state, and emergency situation.
   - The anesthesiologist may call for difficult airway equipment, such as a video laryngoscope or FOB. The learner will be told that there is an anesthesia tech en route with this equipment, but it will be a few minutes

delay, and the OB/GYN surgeon cannot wait that long for induction given the non-reassuring FHR tracing.

- The anesthesiologist should prepare an appropriately sized laryngoscope, oropharyngeal airway (OPA), and nasopharyngeal airway (NPA). The anesthesiologist should consider downsizing the ETT, for instance, to a 6.0 cuffed ETT.
- The anesthesiologist should double-check that suction is working.
- The anesthesiologist may double-check that they have an intubating LMA available in case of inability to bag mask ventilate and inability to intubate.
- The anesthesiologist may attempt to optimize patient positioning for intubation. They may use the levers or head up/down positioning on the bed, or they may use a combination of pillows and blankets, for instance, to optimize the sniffing position.

(b) The OB/GYN surgeon will emergently perform a sterile prep and drape and quickly scrub in for surgery.

(c) The anesthesiologist and OB/GYN surgeon should communicate about when the OB/GYN surgeon is ready to make an incision and when the anesthesiologist can induce anesthesia.

(d) The anesthesiologist should perform a rapid sequence induction and intubation. They may use any combination of medications, such as etomidate, ketamine, or propofol for hypnosis and succinylcholine or rocuronium for muscle relaxation.

4. Phase 3: Difficult airway

(a) The anesthesiologist will induce the patient. They will obtain a grade 4 view by direct laryngoscopy regardless of the choice of laryngoscope and positioning.

(b) The patient will begin to desaturate.

(c) The anesthesiologist will likely attempt to bag mask ventilate the patient. Even with an OPA and/or an NPA, the patient will find it difficult to bag mask ventilate. There will be limited $ETCO_2$ return, limited chest rise, and low tidal volumes. The patient will continue to desaturate.

(d) The anesthesiologist should communicate to the OB/GYN surgeon that they have a difficult airway with an inability to intubate and an inability to bag mask ventilate.

(e) The OB/GYN surgeon and anesthesiologist will likely discuss whether the surgeon can proceed with an emergency cesarean section and deliver the baby, given that the mother is hypoxic and hypercarbic and the baby is likely further compromised by this.

(f) The anesthesiologist should instruct the OB/GYN surgeon to proceed with delivering the baby while the anesthesiologist works to restore ventilation and oxygenation.

(g) The anesthesiologist will likely ask whether the anesthesia technician has arrived yet with the video laryngoscope or FOB. They will be told that the anesthesia technician is in the elevator on their way.

(h) The anesthesiologist should place an LMA. The LMA will seat well, and they will be able to restore oxygenation and ventilation. They will have a good seal with the LMA and achieve good tidal volumes, and oxygenation will improve.

(i) At the same time, the OB/GYN surgeon will quickly deliver the baby and give the baby to the neonatologist. The baby will have low Apgar scores.

5. Phase 4: LMA to ETT conversion
   (a) Shortly after LMA placement, the anesthesia technician will arrive with the video laryngoscope and FOB.
   (b) The anesthesiologist will decide how to convert the LMA for an ETT.
   (c) Given that the patient was difficult to bag mask ventilate, the anesthesiologist will most likely opt to intubate through the LMA using an FOB.
   (d) The anesthesiologist will be easily able to obtain a grade 1 view with assisted jaw thrust and easily pass a 6.0 cuffed ETT over a FOB through the LMA into the trachea.

6. Phase 5: Disposition
   (a) The OB/GYN surgeon will report good uterine tone and normal estimated blood loss. The patient will be doing well hemodynamically and with oxygenation and ventilation.
   (b) The OB/GYN surgeon and anesthesiologist should recap the events and discuss the disposition course.
   (c) They will most likely decide that the patient is stable enough to be extubated and taken to the post-anesthesia care unit (PACU).
   (d) The scenario will end here.

11.6 Anesthesiology Scoring Rubric

Topic: Crash cesarean section with difficult airway		Completed	Not completed
Participants:			
Evaluators:			
Score:			
Tasks		Completed	Not completed
Phase 1: Initial survey			
Communication	Ask surgeons for additional information: Past medical history, history of present illness, current vascular access, resuscitation measures implemented so far, recent labs, and blood products available		
	Ask surgeons about the timing of the cesarean section, specifically the possibility of neuraxial blockade placement versus general anesthesia		
Medical management	Place the patient on full monitors		
	Place the patient on supplemental oxygen		
	Administer fluid bolus and/or pressors		

(continued)

Topic: Crash cesarean section with difficult airway			
Phase 2: Induction			
Communication	Communicate with surgeons about the timing of intubation/surgeon being scrubbed and patient prepped for incision		
Medical management	Pre-oxygenate the patient		
	Call for difficult airway equipment: Video laryngoscope and FOB		
	Prepare intubation equipment: Various sized laryngoscopes, smaller ETTs, OPA, NPA, and LMA.		
	Optimize patient positioning for intubation		
	Perform rapid sequence induction and intubation		
Phase 3: Difficult airway			
Communication	Notify the surgeon of difficult airway		
	Tell the surgeon to proceed with the cesarean section while they continue to try to secure the airway		
	Ask for a status update on the video laryngoscope/FOB being brought to the OR.		
Medical management	Attempt to bag mask ventilate patient		
	Use assistive devices such as OPA and/or NPA to bag mask		
	Recognize difficult airway: Inability to intubate and inability to bag mask ventilate		
	Place an LMA in a timely fashion		
Phase 4: LMA to ETT conversion			
Communication	Notify the surgeon that the airway is secured and the mother's oxygenation and ventilation are improving		
Medical management	Change LMA for ETT. May opt to intubate through LMA using FOB		
Phase 5: Disposition			
Communication	Debrief with surgeons: Airway status, EBL, uterine tone, and hemodynamic stability		
	Discuss with surgeon disposition: Likely extubate and go to PACU		
Medical management	Plan for awake extubation in OR		

Hemorrhagic Shock Due to Uterine Rupture

12

Elsie Bigelow and Claire Sampankanpanich Soria

12.1 Level of Training

- Anesthesiology resident
- Obstetrics/gynecology resident

12.2 Learning Objectives

1. Review the signs and symptoms of uterine rupture.
2. Review management of hemorrhagic shock.
3. Discuss risk factors for uterine rupture.
4. Discuss intraoperative management of uterine rupture and hemorrhage.

12.3 Simulator Environment

1. Location: operating room is located on the labor and delivery floor of a community hospital.
2. Manikin setup:
   (a) Age: high-fidelity birthing manikin capable of cesarean section and vaginal delivery of a neonate manikin.
   (b) Lines: 1 × 20 gauge peripheral intravenous (PIV) line.
3. Medications available:
   (a) Fluids: normal saline, lactated ringers, albumin.

E. Bigelow (✉) · C. S. Soria
University of California, San Diego, San Diego, CA, USA
e-mail: ebigelow@health.ucsd.edu; cssoria@health.ucsd.edu

© The Author(s), under exclusive license to Springer Nature Switzerland AG 2024
C. S. Soria, P. Yao (eds.), *Anesthesiology Simulation*,
https://doi.org/10.1007/978-3-031-80228-7_12

   (b) Blood products: 2 units of packed red blood cells (PRBCs) crossmatched, available upon request, not initially present in the room at the start of the scenario.

   (c) Sedatives/hypnotics: propofol, etomidate, ketamine.

   (d) Paralytics: succinylcholine, rocuronium.

   (e) Cardiac agents: epinephrine, phenylephrine, ephedrine, atropine, vasopressin, norepinephrine, dopamine.

4. Equipment available:

   (a) Airway equipment: face mask, Mapleson, laryngoscope, and cuffed endotracheal tubes (ETTs) of various sizes, stylet, oral airway, nasal trumpet, laryngeal mask airway (LMA), bougie. Video laryngoscopes such as Glidescope or C-MAC and fiberoptic bronchoscopes are available upon request, but there will be a delay.

   (b) Monitors (none on patient initially but will be available upon request): non-invasive blood pressure (NIBP) cuff, 5-lead electrocardiogram (EKG), pulse oximeter, end-tidal carbon dioxide ($ETCO_2$).

   (c) Lines: arterial line kit and transducer, central line kit, PIV kits, available upon request.

   (d) Crash cart with defibrillator, available upon request.

   (e) Trans-esophageal echocardiogram (TEE) and trans-thoracic echocardiogram (TTE) are available upon request.

   (f) Belmont or rapid infuser is available upon request.

12.4 Actors

1. Obstetrics/gynecology team.
2. Anesthesiology team.
3. Bedside nurse/circulator nurse.
4. Scrub technician.
5. Anesthesia technician.

12.5 Case Narrative

1. Background:

   (a) The obstetrician and anesthesiologist are on call at a tertiary care center taking over for the night call shift at 7 pm.

   (b) Background information is to be provided on a piece of paper to the obstetrician only. Please note: this information is not to be given to the anesthesiologist. During the scenario, the obstetrician and anesthesiologist are expected to communicate with each other and relay essential and pertinent information.

     • The patient is a 30-year-old woman, 5′5″, 80 kg, who was admitted this morning at 4 am for induction of labor (IOL) at 39 weeks estimated gestational age (EGA) for gestational diabetes mellitus (GDMA). She is a

> gravid 2 para 1 (G2P1) with a prior delivery 1 year ago at 39 weeks and 4 days EGA via low-transverse cesarean section for arrest of labor. She was deemed a candidate for vaginal birth after cesarean section (VBAC).

- Their current pregnancy has been complicated by GDMA after failing a 3-h blood glucose test, and she has been requiring insulin. The fetus is estimated to be in the 98th percentile for weight. The patient has had three doses of vaginal misoprostol; a Foley bulb was placed at the start of induction but has since been removed. The patient is being augmented with an oxytocin infusion for her labor, and the infusion is currently running at 18 units per hour.

(c) Background information is to be provided on a piece of paper to the anesthesiologist upon request.

- The patient requested an epidural for labor pain this morning at 7 am while at 4 cm dilation. The day shift anesthesiologist placed a single attempt continuous labor epidural at L3/L4, which has been working well since placement. The patient has not had breakthrough pain since epidural placement, and both mother and baby tolerated the procedure well.

12.6 Scenario Development

1. Phase 1: Call to bedside for initial evaluation
   (a) The anesthesiologist receives a page that reads, "Room 1: extreme breakthrough pain despite pushing epidural bolus. Please come assess."
   (b) Upon arrival at the bedside, the anesthesiologist finds whether the patient is writhing in pain with fetal heart rate (FHR) tracing demonstrating recurrent late decelerations and bradycardia to the 110s beats per minute (bpm).
   (c) The anesthesiologist should evaluate the patient by checking vitals via monitor including pulse oximetry (SpO_2), 3-lead or 5-lead EKG, and NIBP cuff.
   (d) Starting vitals will be systolic blood pressure (SBP) low 80s mmHg, SpO_2 98% on room air, and HR 120s sinus tachycardia.
   (e) The anesthesiologist should seek additional patient information about the patient including but not limited to: past medical history, history of labor course, current vascular access, prior epidural functionality, current changes in regards to acute pain, and recent labs.
   (f) Recent labs will be from admission over 12 h ago: white blood cell (WBC) 6, hemoglobin (Hb) 10.5, hematocrit (Hct) 31, platelet (Plt) 120; there is an active type and screen.
   (g) The patient will continue to scream in pain and grab the center of her abdomen, reporting that it started hurting suddenly about 10 min ago and it is the worst her pain has been so far in the course of labor.
   (h) The anesthesiologist should establish a broad differential diagnosis that may include uterine rupture, hemorrhagic shock, malfunctioning epidural and poor pain control, and septic shock.

  (i) The anesthesiologist should recognize the patient's hypotension and tachycardia and the associated fetal distress. Given the patient's hemodynamic instability and fetal distress, the anesthesiologist should call the obstetrician to the bedside emergently for evaluation.

  (j) While waiting for the obstetrician to arrive, the anesthesiologist should stabilize the patient's hemodynamics by administering a fluid bolus, pressors, and supplemental oxygen and repositioning the patient.

  (k) The anesthesiologist may attempt to troubleshoot the epidural, such as by checking the dermatome level of the epidural block; checking the epidural taping on the back and at the insertion site; checking the epidural tubing, bag, and the pump programming; and administering a bolus of local anesthetic by hand with a syringe. All epidural equipment will appear to be functioning normally. The patient will have a bilateral T10 level of decreased sensation to ice on the exam. Bolusing the epidural will improve the patient's pain only minimally.

2. Phase 2: Suspicion for uterine rupture

  (a) The anesthesiologist should have a high suspicion for uterine rupture given the VBAC history, report of a large gestational age fetus, and sudden severe pain not responsive to a functioning epidural.

  (b) Upon arrival at the bedside, the anesthesiologist should communicate to the obstetrician the urgency of the situation, the patient's current status, and their exam findings regarding pain and epidural functionality.

  (c) Focused history and physical exam from the obstetrician will include evaluation of the FHR tracing strips; onset, severity, location, and characterization of the pain; changes in abdominal appearance; signs of bleeding; and cervical exam.

  (d) The obstetrician should discuss with the anesthesiologist what their differential diagnosis is based on the patient's history. There should be clear communication and exchange of pertinent information.

  (e) During the physical examination, the obstetrician will observe new onset vaginal bleeding, increased pain in the upper abdomen, and a cervical exam change consistent with a loss of station.

  (f) The obstetrician should communicate their differential diagnosis with the anesthesiologist, which may include uterine rupture or tachysystole. The team should have a high suspicion of uterine rupture.

3. Phase 3: Management of presumed uterine rupture

  (a) The obstetrician should discontinue the oxytocin infusion and administer terbutaline to the patient to try to stop the uterine contractions and prevent further hemodynamic instability, uterine hypoperfusion, and fetal distress. The terbutaline may be administered subcutaneously, orally, or by inhalation.

  (b) Shortly after terbutaline administration, the FHR tracing originally showing variable decelerations to the 110s will return to a more stable tracing with FHR 140s. The tocometer will show that uterine contractions have stopped.

  (c) The patient will report that the pain has subsided after terbutaline administration.

    (d) The patient's blood pressure and heart rate will improve in response to a 1 L crystalloid bolus, but the patient will remain hypotensive and tachycardic.

    (e) The obstetrician should recognize that the likely etiology is uterine rupture. The obstetrician should decide on an emergent cesarean section and communicate this plan to the anesthesiologist.

4. Phase 4: Emergent cesarean section

    (a) The obstetrician, anesthesiologist, and nurse should move the patient to the operating room for an emergent cesarean section. The obstetrician should notify the charge nurse.

    (b) The anesthesiologist and surgeon should discuss how emergent the cesarean section is. This includes whether there is time to administer a loading bolus in the epidural to do this case under monitored anesthesia care (MAC)/sedation.

    (c) Once the patient is in the operating room, the anesthesiologist and OB/GYN should communicate the urgency of the case based on concern for hemorrhage and current fetal heart tracing.

    (d) The FHR tracing will begin to worsen again with now late decelerations and FHR in the 90s–110s.

    (e) For this simulation scenario, the obstetrician may decide: (a) there is no time to bolus the epidural and request the anesthesiologist to perform this under general anesthesia with endotracheal intubation (GETA); (b) there is limited time, but the anesthesiologist may try to load the epidural very quickly to perform the case under MAC/sedation.

- GETA: The anesthesiologist should optimize patient positioning for intubation; adequately pre-oxygenate the patient; call for an anesthesia technician and difficult airway equipment (various size direct laryngoscopes, endotracheal tubes, video laryngoscope, fiberoptic bronchoscope); perform a rapid sequence induction and intubation after the obstetricians are scrubbed, the patient is prepped and draped, and the obstetrician says it is okay to induce the patient. The choice for induction agents may include propofol, etomidate, or ketamine for hypnotic, and succinylcholine or rocuronium for paralytic. Maintenance of anesthesia should be achieved using a total intravenous anesthetic (TIVA) with minimization of volatile anesthetic to avoid decreased uterine tone. For this simulation scenario, the anesthesiologist will easily obtain a grade 2a view with Mac 3 and be able to pass a 6.0 cuffed ETT successfully without aspiration or desaturation.
- MAC/sedation: The anesthesiologist should only attempt to use the epidural after previously ensuring it is functional. The anesthesiologist should administer a rapid-acting local anesthetic to achieve a T4 level of neuraxial blockade. The choice of local anesthetic may include 3% chloroprocaine. The anesthesiologist should check the level prior to incision, such as by using ice. If at any point it appears the epidural is not functioning or an appropriate level of motor and sensory blockade for cesarean

section has not been achieved, the anesthesiologist should notify the obstetrician and prepare to convert to GETA.

(f) Regardless of the choice of airway management and anesthetic, the anesthesiologist should do the following additional measures:

- Call for blood products to be brought to the room. This may include 1–2 units of PRBCs. They may call for uncrossmatched blood or send an additional laboratory sample for type and cross.
- Establish additional intravascular access. The anesthesiologist will likely place a second large-bore PIV. As the case progresses, the anesthesiologist may opt to place a radial arterial line for frequent blood draws and closer hemodynamic monitoring. The anesthesiologist may also opt to place a central line if they plan to start a massive transfusion or pressors/inotropes later on in the case.
- Administer fluids (crystalloids, colloids), pressors/inotropes, and blood products as needed based on surgical blood loss and hemodynamic instability. The patient will remain hypotensive and tachycardic but responsive to fluids and pressors.

5. Phase 5: Hemorrhagic shock

(a) The obstetrician will start the incision uneventfully and notice upon entry into the abdomen that the uterus has ruptured. The baby will be delivered uneventfully and handed off to the neonatal intensive care unit (NICU) team. The obstetrician should communicate with the anesthesiologist the finding of a ruptured uterus.

(b) The placenta will be removed without difficulty, but the obstetrician will observe profuse bleeding from the uterus and poor uterine tone.

(c) The patient will remain hypotensive and tachycardic.

(d) The anesthesiologist should continue supportive measures including blood transfusion, volume resuscitation, and pressors.

(e) The anesthesiologist will likely place an arterial line and send an arterial blood gas (ABG) or at least a venous blood gas (VBG) from a PIV.

(f) The anesthesiologist and surgeon should discuss the current status: estimated blood loss, the status of surgical hemostasis, pressors/fluids/blood products given so far, current vital signs, and recent labs.

(g) ABG will be notable for metabolic acidosis, anemia, and hypocalcemia.

(h) The obstetrician will continue to struggle to obtain surgical hemostasis.

(i) The obstetrician should communicate whether they need specific hemorrhagic medications such as oxytocin, methylergonovine (methergine), carboprost tromethamine (hemabate), misoprostol, and tranexamic acid (TXA).

6. Phase 6: Stability and disposition

(a) As the team together continues supportive measures, the patient will become more stable: adequate surgical hemostasis, improved hemodynamics, and weaning off of pressors.

(b) The OB/GYN and anesthesiologist should recap the events and current state of the resuscitation. This will include the status of hemodynamic stability and recent labs.

(c) Together the OB/GYN and anesthesiologist should discuss the disposition of the patient. If the patient is intubated, they may decide to extubate the patient with transfer of care to a monitored bed for closer monitoring or keep the patient intubated and sedated with transport to the intensive care unit.

(d) The scenario will end here.

12.7   Anesthesiology Scoring Rubric

Topic: Hemorrhagic shock due to uterine rupture		Completed	Not completed
Participants:			
Evaluators:			
Score:			
Tasks		Completed	Not completed
Phase 1: Call to bedside for initial evaluation			
Communication	Perform focused history and physical: Pertinent past medical history, history of labor course, current vascular access, prior epidural functionality, and current changes in regards to acute pain; recent labs. Call the obstetrician to discuss the case and differential diagnoses.		
Medical management	Place the patient on full monitors. Stabilize hemodynamics with fluid bolus, pressors, supplemental oxygen, and repositioning. Attempts to troubleshoot the labor epidural: Check tubing/pump, sensory blockade level, may hand bolus with a short-acting, rapid-onset local anesthetic. Formulate a differential diagnosis for the etiology of severe breakthrough pain.		
Phase 2: Suspicion for uterine rupture			
Communication	Communicate with obstetrician suspicion for uterine rupture given VBAC, large for gestational age (LGA) fetus, and severe pain unresponsive to functioning epidural.		
Medical management	Continue supportive care of the patient.		
Phase 3: Management of presumed uterine rupture			
Communication	Remain in regular communication with the obstetrician about changes in exam/stability. Discuss the level of urgency of cesarean section based on the degree of bleeding and FHR tracing.		
Medical management	Continue to provide supportive measures. Begin contacting additional staff (anesthesia tech, backup anesthesiologist) about preparing the operating room (OR) for a possible emergency C-section.		

(continued)

Topic: Hemorrhagic shock due to uterine rupture			
Phase 4: Emergent cesarean section			
Communication	Discuss the timing of the C-section, namely if there is time to load the epidural versus induce general anesthesia.		
Medical management	If GETA: Perform rapid sequence induction/intubation.		
	If MAC/sedation: After assuring a functioning epidural, administer a hand bolus of rapid-acting local anesthetic via epidural.		
	Call for blood products to OR.		
	Establish additional intravascular access (large-bore IV, arterial line, and/or central access) as indicated.		
	Administer fluids, pressors/inotropes, and blood products as needed.		
Phase 5: Hemorrhagic shock			
Communication	Remain in regular communication with the obstetrician about patient stability, surgical hemostasis, and blood loss.		
Medical management	Escalate fluid resuscitation, transfusion, and pressors/inotropes.		
	Administer hemorrhage medications in a timely fashion.		
	Send frequent ABGs or VBGs to guide resuscitation.		
	Send additional labs such as thromboelastogram. (TEG), coagulation panel, complete blood count (CBC), and lactate.		
Phase 6: Stability and disposition			
Communication	Debrief with obstetricians: Current hemodynamic stability, estimated blood loss (EBL), most recent labs, blood products given, and status of resuscitation.		
	Discuss disposition planning of the patient following OR including whether to remain intubated.		
Medical management	If choosing to remain intubated, transport to the ICU for further evaluation and care.		
	If hemodynamically stable and agreed by the team, transport to post-anesthesia care unit (PACU) for further evaluation and care.		

High Spinal Block in Obstetrics

Elsie Bigelow and Claire Sampankanpanich Soria

13.1 Level of Training

- Anesthesiology resident
- Obstetrics/gynecology resident

13.2 Learning Objectives

1. Review the signs and symptoms of high spinal block
2. Review the management of fetal bradycardia

13.3 Simulator Environment

1. Location: operating room (OR) located on the labor and delivery floor of a community hospital.
2. Manikin setup:
   (a) Age: high-fidelity birthing manikin capable of cesarean section and vaginal delivery of a neonate manikin.
   (b) Lines: 1 × 20-gauge peripheral intravenous (PIV) line.
3. Medications available:
   (a) Fluids: normal saline, lactated Ringer's solution, and albumin.
   (b) Blood products: 2 units of packed red blood cells (PRBCs) crossmatched, available upon request, and not initially present in the room at the start of the scenario.
   (c) Sedatives/hypnotics: propofol, etomidate, and ketamine.

E. Bigelow (✉) · C. S. Soria
University of California, San Diego, San Diego, CA, USA
e-mail: ebigelow@health.ucsd.edu; cssoria@health.ucsd.edu

© The Author(s), under exclusive license to Springer Nature Switzerland AG 2024
C. S. Soria, P. Yao (eds.), *Anesthesiology Simulation*,
https://doi.org/10.1007/978-3-031-80228-7_13

   (d) Paralytics: succinylcholine and rocuronium.

   (e) Cardiac agents: epinephrine, phenylephrine, ephedrine, atropine, vasopressin, norepinephrine, and dopamine.

4. Equipment available:

   (a) Airway equipment: face mask, Mapleson, laryngoscopes and cuffed endotracheal tubes (ETTs) of various sizes, stylet, oral airway, nasal trumpet, laryngeal mask airway (LMA), and bougie. Video laryngoscopes such as GlideScope or C-MAC and fiberoptic bronchoscope are available upon request, but there will be a delay.

   (b) Monitors (none on patient initially but will be available upon request): non-invasive blood pressure (NIBP) cuff, 5-lead electrocardiogram (EKG), pulse oximeter, and end-tidal carbon dioxide ($ETCO_2$).

   (c) Lines: arterial line kit and transducer, central line kit, and PIV kits, available upon request.

   (d) Crash cart with defibrillator, available upon request.

   (e) Trans-esophageal echocardiogram (TEE) and trans-thoracic echocardiogram (TTE) are available upon request.

   (f) Belmont or rapid infuser, available upon request.

13.4 Actors

1. Obstetrics/gynecology team
2. Anesthesiology team
3. Bedside nurse/circulator nurse
4. Scrub technician
5. Anesthesia technician
6. Neonatal intensive care unit (NICU) team

13.5 Case Narrative

1. Background:

   (a) The obstetrician and anesthesiologist are working together overnight at a tertiary care center.

   (b) Background information is to be provided on a piece of paper to the obstetrician only. Please note that this information is not to be given to the anesthesiologist. During the scenario, the obstetrician and anesthesiologist are expected to communicate with each other and relay essential and pertinent information.

     • The patient is a 28-year-old woman, with a height of 5′2″ and a weight of 75 kg, who was sent in from an outpatient clinic due to elevated blood pressure of 162/94 to rule out pre-eclampsia. She is a gravid 1 para 0 (G1P0) and at 38 weeks of estimated gestational age (EGA) with no medical problems throughout this pregnancy. Upon presentation to triage, the patient's first blood pressure was 160/88 and second blood pressure 15 min later was 164/92. Her blood pressure was treated with labetalol, and the decision was made to admit the patient for an induction of labor.

- Labs were sent upon admission, including complete blood count (CBC), complete metabolic panel (CMP), and protein-to-creatine ratio (P:C ratio). Results of laboratory studies include a P:C ratio of 0.4, platelets of 198, hemoglobin (hgb) of 11.5, and aspartate aminotransferase (AST)/alanine aminotransferase (ALT) within normal limits. She was given a magnesium bolus, and an infusion was started according to hospital protocol. The patient has had three doses of vaginal misoprostol; a Foley bulb was placed at the start of induction but has since been removed. The patient is being augmented with an oxytocin infusion for her labor, and the infusion is currently running at 10 units per hour.

(c) Background information is to be provided on a piece of paper to the anesthesiologist upon request.

- The patient requested an epidural for labor pain this evening at 12 pm while at 3-cm dilation. Upon review of the chart, the patient is a 28-year-old woman, weighing 75 kg, G1P0, and at 38 weeks of EGA. She is admitted for induction of labor due to severe pre-eclampsia. The patient has platelets of 198, hgb of 11.5, and a most recent blood pressure of 130/68 and is currently on a magnesium infusion.
- The daytime anesthesiologist signed out that the epidural has been slightly patchy and they have had to give multiple boluses of 0.125% bupivacaine during the last few hours.

13.6   Scenario Development

1. Phase 1: Call for urgent C-section
   (a) The anesthesiologist receives a page that reads, "Room for urgent C-section due to recurrent fetal decelerations."
   (b) The anesthesiologist should discuss the urgency versus emergency status of the C-section. The obstetrics team says it's urgent and needs to go to the OR as soon as possible, but not emergent.
   (c) The anesthesiologist should briefly review the record and evaluate the patient, including a recent blood pressure from a NIBP cuff, a pulse oximetry reading (SpO$_2$), and heart rate (HR). The anesthesiologist should seek additional patient information about the patient, including, but not limited to, past medical history, history of labor course, current vascular access, and recent labs.
   (d) In addition, the anesthesiologist should go to bedside to evaluate the current dermatomal level of the epidural. The dermatomal level will be at the T12 level.
2. Phase 2: Trial of loading the epidural of C-section

(a) The anesthesiologist should place the patient on appropriate monitors, including NIBP, SpO_2, and HR monitoring, and ensure the baby is also on the fetal monitor.

(b) The baseline pre-procedure NIBP is 134/78, SpO_2 is 98%, and HR is 78. Fetal heart tracing demonstrates a baseline of 130 beats per minute.

(c) The anesthesiologist should load the epidural catheter with either lidocaine or chloroprocaine. Despite bolusing the catheter with a local anesthetic, the dermatomal level of the block will not rise beyond T12.

(d) The anesthesiologist will opt to convert from an epidural block to a spinal block. The anesthesiologist can perform either a single-shot spinal or a combined spinal epidural.

3. Phase 3: Suspicion for high spinal block

(a) Immediately after lying down, the patient begins to report she is feeling very lightheaded, dizzy, nauseous, and short of breath.

(b) The anesthesiologist should cycle the NIBP and find the blood pressure to be 60/40. Vasopressor support should be initiated.

(c) Immediately, the anesthesiologist should check the dermatome level of the spinal block. Regardless of the dose of local anesthetic, the patient now has evidence of a high spinal.

(d) The anesthesiologist should continue to cycle the blood pressure frequently and get prepared for supportive measures, including further vasopressor support and possible airway support.

(e) The obstetrician should discuss with the anesthesiologist the current scenario. Together, they must communicate the circumstances of severe hypotension following the recent replacement of a spinal anesthetic.

(f) The anesthesiologist should take diagnostic steps to identify the height of the spinal. They may check a level with ice or have the patient squeeze the anesthesiologist's hand for a strength test.

4. Phase 4: Fetal deceleration and crash C-section.

(a) Despite vasopressor support and patient repositioning, the fetus begins to have severe bradycardia to the 40s.

(b) The obstetric team decides to do a crash C-section, splashes iodine onto the abdomen, and quickly prepares the patient. The obstetric team calls for the NICU team to emergently come to the OR for fetal resuscitation.

- If the simulation team creates a scenario where the spinal continues to rise and the patient develops apnea, the anesthesiologist will have to emergently intubate and ventilate the patient.
- If the simulation team has the spinal stop rising before airway compromise, the C-section will proceed under neuraxial anesthesia alone.

(c) The obstetric team will promptly deliver the baby, deliver the placenta, and achieve hemostasis.

5. Phase 5: Stability and disposition

(a) The obstetric team closes the incision from emergent cesarean delivery. The anesthesiologist continues to support the patient if either under general anesthesia or under neuraxial blockade.

(b) The team together continues supportive measures, and the patient will become more stable: adequate surgical hemostasis and improved hemodynamics.

(c) Together, the obstetric and anesthesiology teams decide to transfer the patient to the recovery area following a crash C-section.

(d) The scenario will end here.

13.7 Anesthesiology Scoring Rubric

Topic: High spinal block in obstetrics		Completed	Not completed
Participants:			
Evaluators:			
Score:			
Tasks		Completed	Not completed
Phase 1: Call for urgent C-section			
Communication	Perform a focused history and physical examination: Pertinent past medical history, history of labor course, current vascular access, prior epidural functionality, and current changes in regard to acute pain; recent labs		
	Call the obstetrician to discuss the urgency versus emergency nature of surgery		
Medical management	Evaluate the current dermatomal level of the epidural		
Phase 2: Trial of loading the epidural of C-section			
Communication	Communicate with the obstetrician to plan to utilize the existing epidural catheter		
Medical management	Place the patient on appropriate monitors, including NIBP, SpO_2, and EKG		
	Load the epidural catheter with either lidocaine or chloroprocaine and evaluate the anticipated rising dermatomal level		
	Convert from an epidural block to a spinal block with either a single-shot spinal or a combined spinal epidural		
Phase 3: Suspicion for high spinal block			
Communication	Discuss with the obstetric team concern for the high spinal block		
Medical management	Provide supportive measures for hypotension, including fluids and vasopressors		
	Evaluate the level of spinal with ice and with neuro-examination via upper extremity neuro-examination		
Phase 4: Fetal deceleration and crash C-section			
Communication	Discuss fetal heart rate and necessity for an emergency C-section		
	If the airway compromises with the level of spinal, communicate the need to intubate and convert to general anesthesia prior to incision		

(continued)

Topic: High spinal block in obstetrics			
Medical management	If general endotracheal anesthesia (GETA) performs rapid sequence induction/intubation		
	If the spinal does not inhibit airway integrity, continue with supportive measures for the high spinal block		
	Establish additional intravascular access (large bore IV, arterial line, and/or central access) as indicated		
	Administer fluids, pressors/inotropes, and blood products as needed		
Phase 5: Stability and disposition			
Communication	Remain in regular communication with the obstetrician about patient stability, surgical hemostasis, and blood loss		
Medical management	Continue supportive measures while under general anesthesia or spinal block		
	Administer hemorrhage medications in a timely fashion if needed		
	If hemodynamically stable and agreed by the team, transport to post-anesthesia care unit (PACU) for further evaluation and care		

Eclampsia

14

Caitlin Krol and Claire Sampankanpanich Soria

14.1 Level of Training

- Anesthesiology resident
- Obstetrics/gynecology resident

14.2 Learning Objectives

1. Review the signs and symptoms of preeclampsia.
2. Review the signs and symptoms of eclampsia.
3. Understand the systemic effects of severe preeclampsia and the complications that can arise.
4. Discuss intraoperative management of preeclampsia that evolves into eclampsia.

14.3 Simulator Environment

1. Location: main operating room of a tertiary care center on the obstetric floor.
2. Manikin setup:
    (a) Age: adult.
    (b) Lines: 1 × 20 gauge peripheral intravenous (PIV) line in L forearm.
3. Medications available:
    (a) Fluids: normal saline, lactated ringers, albumin.
    (b) Blood products: available upon request.
    (c) Sedatives/hypnotics: propofol, etomidate, midazolam, fentanyl.
    (d) Paralytics: succinylcholine, rocuronium.

C. Krol (✉) · C. S. Soria
University of California, San Diego, San Diego, CA, USA
e-mail: ckrol@health.ucsd.edu; cssoria@health.ucsd.edu

© The Author(s), under exclusive license to Springer Nature Switzerland AG 2024
C. S. Soria, P. Yao (eds.), *Anesthesiology Simulation*,
https://doi.org/10.1007/978-3-031-80228-7_14

    (e) Cardiac agents: epinephrine, phenylephrine, ephedrine, atropine, vasopressin, norepinephrine, dopamine, labetalol, esmolol, nitroglycerin.

    (f) OB-specific medications: magnesium sulfate, oxytocin, carboprost, and methylergonovine.

4. Equipment available:

    (a) Airway equipment: Code bag [including mask, Mapleson, laryngoscope, and cuffed endotracheal tube (ETTs) of various sizes, stylet, oral airway, nasal trumpet, laryngeal mask airway (LMA), bougie]. Video laryngoscopes such as Glidescope or C-MAC and fiberoptic bronchoscopes are available upon request, but there will be a delay.

    (b) Monitors (none on patient initially but will be available upon request): non-invasive blood pressure (NIBP) cuff, 5-lead electrocardiogram (EKG), pulse oximeter (SpO_2) , end-tidal carbon dioxide ($ETCO_2$).

    (c) Lines (available upon request): arterial line kit and transducer, central line kit, PIV kits.

    (d) Crash cart with defibrillator.

    (e) Trans-esophageal echocardiogram (TEE) and trans-thoracic echocardiogram TTE) are available upon request.

14.4 Actors

1. Obstetrics/gynecology team.
2. Anesthesia team.
3. Circulator nurse.
4. Scrub technician.
5. Anesthesia technician.

14.5 Case Narrative

1. Background:

    (a) The OB/GYN surgeon and anesthesiologist are on call at a tertiary care center.

    (b) The anesthesiologist receives a page that reads, "STAT C-section to OR 1 due to fetal distress."

- Upon arrival in the OR, they will note that the patient is an obese 37-year-old woman who came in through the emergency department (ED) in labor. Her airway exam is a Mallampati 3 with a normal mouth opening, normal thyromental distance, and a large neck circumference. She has one 20 G PIV in the left forearm. She is extremely anxious, tearful, and in distress.

    (c) The OB/GYN surgeon will have additional information about the patient, provided to them on a sheet of paper for the scenario. The surgeon and anesthesiologist will need to speak with each other to share this information.

(d) Background information is to be provided on a piece of paper to the OB/GYN surgeon only. The team will need to have an adequate signout to get all of the information provided.
- The patient is an obese 37-year-old female G3P2 at approximately 35 weeks with minimal prenatal care and an unknown past medical history (PMH). No known drug allergies. Does not take any medications at home. Labs were drawn downstairs in the ED and pending. On fetal monitoring, the team started to see recurrent late decelerations with minimal variability, which is why a STAT C-section has been called.
- The patient was refusing additional monitors in the ED as she was inconsolable and the "blood pressure cuff was too tight." The only vitals recorded were upon EMS arrival: SpO_2 96%, heart rate (HR) 100, BP 160/100. She continues to complain of a "bad headache" which started yesterday and her "puffy legs."

2. Phase 1: Initial survey
   (a) The anesthesiologist should place the patient on full monitors, including SpO_2, NIBP, and 5-lead EKG.
   (b) Starting vital signs will be systolic blood pressure (SBP) 160s mmHg, SpO_2 95% on room air, and HR 110s sinus tachycardia.
   (c) The anesthesiologist should expeditiously seek additional information about the patient, including past medical history, history of present illness (HPI), home medications, allergies, last food or drink, current vascular access, treatment measures implemented so far, recent labs, blood products, and medications ordered/available. They may try to obtain this information by interviewing the patient, reviewing the electronic medical record, and speaking with the obstetrician.
   (d) The obstetrician should provide the information they have to the anesthesiologist in a timely fashion. They should have already ordered anti-hypertensive medications and a magnesium infusion at this point. These steps should be confirmed with the team.
   (e) The obstetrician should voice their concerns about the patient (given the history that they know thus far) and their plan to deliver the fetus as quickly as possible given the recurrent decelerations on fetal heart rate (FHR) tracing.

3. Phase 2: Induction and intubation
   (a) Preparation:
   - The anesthesiologist should communicate with the obstetrician about recommendations or plans such as:
     - How they want to move forward with the case, namely whether it will be under general anesthesia with endotracheal intubation versus MAC with a neuraxial block (spinal versus epidural).
     - Additional vascular access that they may need (e.g., large-bore PIV) and invasive monitors (e.g., arterial line).
     - Additional medications such as anti-hypertensives, hemorrhage medications, and whether to continue magnesium sulfate intraoperatively.
     - The risk of bleeding and the need for blood products and hemorrhage medications like carboprost, methylergonovine, and tranexamic acid.

If the anesthesiologist does want additional vascular access, they should clearly communicate whether they want this done before or after induction, as the obstetrician may request to start the cesarean section first.

- A type and screen will have been sent in the ED but not a type and cross. Should the anesthesiologist call for blood products? In the simulation scenario, there will be a delayed arrival.
- The anesthesiologist may also prepare inotropes and pressors as boluses or infusions. They should anticipate significant hypotension after induction of anesthesia in the setting of pre-eclampsia.
- Given that the team does not have lab results yet, it is reasonable to assume that the patient has severe pre-eclampsia. Evidence for this includes two documented high blood pressures in the severe range and evidence of end-organ dysfunction (headache, peripheral edema).
- The anesthesiologist will likely opt for a general anesthetic rather than a neuraxial block given the risk of thrombocytopenia, platelet dysfunction, and potential hematoma with attempted neuraxial block placement.

(b) Note: If the anesthesiologist intends to perform any of these steps prior to induction, they should name a brief timeframe in which to achieve these tasks. The OB/GYN surgeon and anesthesiologist should balance these goals with the urgency of beginning surgery to deliver the fetus as soon as possible.

(c) Induction

- As the team is getting ready to induce, the patient will become inconsolable and altered. She mumbles that she is not feeling well, and she will then lose consciousness and start seizing. Vitals at this time will show SpO_2 92%, HR 120s, and BP 170s/110s. The FHR will show bradycardia into the 80s with minimal variability.
- The anesthesiologist should administer medications to terminate the seizure. The most readily available medication in the OR would be midazolam, a short-acting benzodiazepine, intravenously, or propofol.
- The anesthesiologist should support the airway by administering 100% FiO_2 via a full face mask and proceed with rapid sequence induction and intubation to minimize aspiration risk and restore adequate oxygenation and ventilation.
- The seizure should be identified quickly, and an obstetrician should be notified. The interventions should be communicated to the obstetrician in a timely fashion. The obstetrician should communicate how they intend to proceed, most likely an emergency or crash C-section.

(d) Intubation

- The anesthesiologist will likely induce with propofol and succinylcholine. The intubation will proceed uneventfully. The anesthesiologist will encounter a grade 1 view with notable edema but be able to pass a 6.0 cuffed endotracheal tube easily. No aspiration will occur if the anesthesiologist proceeds quickly.

   (e) Incision
- The anesthesiologist may tell the obstetrician to proceed with incision and delivery of the baby as they are inducing or opt to wait until after the airway is secured. Either choice is acceptable, given the patient had started seizing and presumably the baby also became more unstable.

   (f) After induction, labs sent from the ED will result in Hb 10, WBC 12, plt 65, AST 96, ALT 98, and serum CR 1.3.

   (g) If the anesthesiologist opts to do point-of-care glucose intraoperatively, fingerstick glucose will be 120.

4. Phase 3: Delivery and hemorrhage

   (a) The fetus will be delivered expeditiously with poor Appearance, Pulse, Grimace, Activity, and Respiration (APGAR) scores. The fetus will be handed off to the neonatal intensive care unit (NICU) team to be resuscitated.

   (b) Magnesium should be infused (pending that the BP is stable at this point).

   (c) The anesthesiologist should opt to run a total intravenous anesthetic (TIVA) such as a propofol infusion, rather than a volatile anesthetic, to help with uterine tone.

   (d) Oxytocin bolus should be given, and an infusion started.

   (e) The obstetrician will notice that the uterine tone is poor. They reveal that it is a "very boggy uterus." They will ask to give another uterotonic. Methylergonovine should not be administered at this time given the patient's severe pre-eclampsia.

   (f) The obstetrician will be able to obtain better surgical control of bleeding, but the patient will become increasingly tachycardic and hypotensive.

   (g) If alternative IV access and the arterial line were not done at the beginning of the case due to the emergent nature of the delivery, the anesthesiologist should consider getting large-bore IV access at this time as well as an arterial line.

   (h) The anesthesiologist should send labs, such as a venous blood gas (VBG) or, if they place an arterial line, an arterial blood gas (ABG).
- Blood gas will show anemia (Hb 8) and metabolic acidosis (pH 7.25, $PaCO_2$ 35, PaO_2 200, HCO_3 19).
- The anesthesiologist should recognize this and continue volume resuscitation as well as call for blood products to be brought to the OR.
- The anesthesiologist should communicate regularly and at appropriate decision-making points, such as deciding to transfuse blood and inquiring about uterine tone, surgical control of bleeding, and estimated blood loss (surveying the surgical field, checking the suction canisters, drapes, wet laps, etc.).

   (i) If the patient is not resuscitated appropriately (i.e., inadequately balanced blood product transfusion, lack of correction of electrolyte abnormalities, etc.), then the patient will code (this will be up to the simulator instructor's discretion), and advanced cardiac life support (ACLS) will need to be started by the anesthesiologist.

(j) If a thromboelastogram (TEG) was ordered, it would reveal a prolonged R time, K time, and decreased alpha angle, consistent with hypo-coagulopathy.

5. Phase 4: Hypoxia
   (a) As the team continues these supportive measures, the patient's hemodynamics will eventually improve.
   (b) Surgical hemostasis will be achieved.
   (c) However, oxygen saturation will remain in the low 90s on 100% FiO_2. ABG will show a relatively low PaO_2 for a high FiO_2.
      - A chest X-ray should be considered. If completed, it will show bilateral pulmonary infiltrates.
      - The anesthesiologist should recognize the low P-to-F ratio is indicative of moderate to severe acute respiratory distress syndrome (ARDS).
      - The anesthesiologist should survey the ventilator and circuit; manually bag to assess compliance; and auscultate breath sounds. Compliance will be ok, but the anesthesiologist will auscultate bilateral crackles.
      - The team should have a high suspicion of pulmonary edema in the setting of eclampsia, large-volume resuscitation, and blood transfusion.
      - The anesthesiologist should adjust ventilator settings to try to improve oxygenation, such as raising the positive end expiratory pressure (PEEP). They may consider diuretics intraoperatively pending hemodynamic stability and weaning of pressors.

6. Phase 5: Disposition
   (a) The patient will require the continuation of low-dose pressors and continue to have hypotension and tachycardia without them.
   (b) Repeat ABGs will demonstrate worsening and then improving metabolic acidosis and anemia, but continued hypoxia with a low PaO_2 to FiO_2 ratio.
   (c) The obstetrician and anesthesiologist should recap the events of the severe preeclampsia that evolved into eclampsia and how it was treated. They should discuss the current state of the resuscitation. This will include a status update on hemodynamic stability, recent labs (e.g., anemia, metabolic acidosis, and hypoxemia), and medications (what was given during the case and what pressors/inotropes the pressor is on currently).
   (d) The obstetrician and anesthesiologist should discuss disposition postoperatively. Given the patient's continued hypoxia and pressor requirement, the patient should remain intubated and taken to the surgical intensive care unit (SICU).
   (e) The team may decide to go to the CT scanner en route to the SICU to obtain a CT head, given the patient had a seizure, remains intubated, and cannot participate in a neurological exam at this time.
   (f) The scenario will end with the decision to transport to the ICU.

Anesthesiology Scoring Rubric

Topic: Preeclampsia to eclampsia		Completed	Not completed
Participants:			
Evaluators:			
Score:			
Tasks			
Phase 1: Initial survey			
Communication	Obtain additional information in a timely fashion: PMH, medications, HPI, nil per os (NPO), IV access, medications/interventions so far.		
	Discuss with the obstetrician the urgency of C-section, FHR tracing, and timing/safety of general anesthesia (GA) with ETT vs. neuraxial block.		
Medical management	Place standard monitors and identify severe range blood pressure.		
	Consider establishing additional IV access and an arterial line. May also place post-induction.		
	Administer magnesium infusion for seizure prophylaxis.		
Phase 2: Induction and intubation			
Communication	Discuss with the obstetrician the pros/cons of general anesthesia with endotracheal tube (GETA) vs. neuraxial block.		
	Discuss the plan for blood products and hemorrhage medications like uterotonics.		
	Notify obstetrician immediately of seizure, progression to eclampsia.		
	Communicate with the obstetrician about the timing of induction and intubation.		
	Communicate with the obstetrician about the timing of the incision and delivery of the fetus.		
Medical management	Identify the seizure.		
	Treat the seizure immediately (e.g., midazolam or propofol).		
	Secure the airway in a timely fashion (100% FiO_2 via bag-mask ventilation initially).		
	Perform a rapid sequence induction and intubation.		
	Place arterial labs and send rainbow labs (e.g., complete blodo count (CBC), basic metabolic panel (BMP), coags, and ABG).		
	Consider differential diagnosis for seizure besides eclampsia (e.g., hypoglycemia).		
Phase 3: Delivery and hemorrhage			
Communication	Remain in regular communication with the obstetrician about uterine tone, estimated blood loss, and surgical hemostasis.		
	Update the obstetrician at appropriate points about blood transfusion, pressor requirements, and hemodynamic stability.		

(continued)

Topic: Preeclampsia to eclampsia			
Medical management	Maintain anesthesia using a TIVA to improve uterine tone.		
	Administer oxytocin after delivery.		
	Administer hemorrhage medications and uterotonics in coordination with the obstetrician.		
	Place additional IV access and arterial line.		
	Send frequent repeat ABGs.		
	Identify anemia and uncontrolled hemorrhage.		
	Transfuse blood products judiciously.		
	Identify metabolic acidosis on ABG.		
	Identify hypotension and tachycardia.		
	Administer pressors and inotropes titrated to hemodynamics.		
Phase 4: Hypoxia			
Communication	Notify the surgeon about hypoxia.		
	Review differential diagnosis with surgeon, including pulmonary edema and ARDS in the setting of eclampsia.		
Medical management	Identify hypoxia, including low SpO_2 and low PaO_2.		
	Recognize low PaO_2 to FiO_2 ratio and presence of moderate-severe ARDS.		
	Establish differential diagnosis for hypoxia, including pulmonary edema.		
	Survey ventilator, circuit, check compliance, and auscultate breath sounds.		
	May obtain intraoperative chest X-ray.		
	Adjust ventilator settings in response to suspected pulmonary edema and ARDS.		
Phase 5: Disposition			
Communication	Debrief with surgeons: Preeclampsia that evolved to eclampsia, complicated by moderate-severe ARDS/pulmonary edema.		
	Discuss disposition planning: Remain intubated to SICU, possible head CT en route to SICU.		
	Review the current status of resuscitation: Blood products, labs, pressor requirement, and ventilator/oxygen requirements.		
Medical management	Keep the patient intubated given ongoing ARDS, hypoxia, and hemodynamic instability.		
	Consider head CT given recent seizure and remaining intubated.		
	Identify patient needs ICU level care.		

Amniotic Fluid Embolism

15

Claire Sampankanpanich Soria

15.1　Level of Training

- Anesthesiology resident
- Obstetrics/gynecology resident

15.2　Learning Objectives

1. Review the signs and symptoms of amniotic fluid embolism (AFE).
2. Review risk factors for the occurrence of AFE.
3. Discuss intraoperative management of AFE.

15.3　Simulator Environment

1. Location: main operating room (OR) of a tertiary care center.
2. Manikin setup:
    (a) Age: adult.
    (b) Lines: 1 × 20 gauge peripheral intravenous (PIV) line.
3. Medications available:
    (a) Fluids: normal saline, lactated ringers, albumin.
    (b) Blood products: 2 units of packed red blood cells (PRBCs).
    (c) Sedatives/hypnotics: propofol, etomidate.
    (d) Paralytics: succinylcholine, rocuronium.
    (e) Cardiac agents: epinephrine, phenylephrine, ephedrine, atropine, vasopressin, norepinephrine, dopamine.

C. S. Soria (✉)
University of California, San Diego, San Diego, CA, USA
e-mail: cssoria@health.ucsd.edu

4. Equipment available:
   (a) Airway equipment: face mask, Mapleson, laryngoscope, and cuffed endotracheal tube (ETTs) of various sizes, stylet, oral airway, nasal trumpet, laryngeal mask airway (LMA), bougie. Video laryngoscopes such as Glidescope or C-MAC and fiberoptic bronchoscopes are available upon request, but there will be a delay.
   (b) Monitors (none on patient initially but will be available upon request): noninvasive blood pressure (NIBP) cuff, 5-lead electrocardiogram (EKG), pulse oximeter, end-tidal carbon dioxide ($ETCO_2$).
   (c) Lines (available upon request): arterial line kit and transducer, central line kit, PIV kits.
   (d) Crash cart with defibrillator.
   (e) Trans-esophageal echocardiogram (TEE) and trans-thoracic echocardiogram TTE) are available upon request.

15.4 Actors

1. Obstetrics/gynecology team
2. Anesthesia team
3. Circulator nurse
4. Scrub technician
5. Anesthesia technician

15.5 Case Narrative

1. Background:
   (a) The OB/GYN surgeon and anesthesiologist are on call at a tertiary care center.
   (b) The anesthesiologist receives a page that reads, "Level 1 dilation and evacuation."
       - Upon arrival in the OR, they will note that the patient is a 38-year-old woman, with a normal BMI, who is otherwise healthy, has a reassuring airway exam, has one 20 G PIV in the hand, and is currently receiving 1 unit of PRBCs that is programmed to infuse over 1 h on a pump. She appears pale and lethargic.
   (c) The OB/GYN surgeon will have additional information about the patient, provided to them on a sheet of paper for the scenario. The surgeon and anesthesiologist will need to speak with each other to share this information.
   (d) Background information is to be provided on a piece of paper to the OB/GYN surgeon only. This is not to be given to the anesthesiologist.
       - The patient was admitted overnight. She is 22 weeks pregnant. This is her first pregnancy, and it is an undesired pregnancy. She recently underwent

an attempted dilation and evacuation at Planned Parenthood. However, there was excessive bleeding, so she was transferred to this tertiary care hospital for a higher level of care.

- The patient continued to bleed more heavily overnight. Hemoglobin on admission was 10.5 g/dL. A repeat complete blood count (CBC) was drawn and sent and is still pending. The primary team ordered 1 U PRBC for transfusion. The patient was typed and crossmatched for 2 U PRBCs. The second unit is in the blood bank.

2. Phase 1: Initial survey
   (a) The anesthesiologist should place the patient on full monitors, including pulse oximetry (SpO$_2$), NIBP, and 5-lead EKG.
   (b) Starting vital signs will be systolic blood pressure (SBP) 90s mmHg, SpO$_2$ 98% on room air, and heart rate (HR) 120s sinus tachycardia.
   (c) The anesthesiologist should seek additional information about the patient, including past medical history, history of present illness, current vascular access, resuscitation measures implemented so far, recent labs, blood products available, current estimated blood loss (EBL), predicted additional blood loss, and source of the bleed. They may try to obtain this information by interviewing the patient, reviewing the electronic medical record, and speaking with the OB/GYN surgeon.
   (d) The OB/GYN surgeon should provide the information they have to the anesthesiologist in a timely fashion.
   (e) The OB/GYN should establish expectations about how much blood loss is anticipated and keep the anesthesiologist informed about blood loss, coagulopathy, or other complications.

3. Phase 2: Induction and intubation
   (a) The anesthesiologist should communicate with the OB/GYN surgeon about recommendations or plans for additional vascular access (e.g., large-bore PIV), invasive monitors (e.g., arterial line), and blood products. They should state whether they want to place these prior to induction or after induction.
   (b) The anesthesiologist may call the blood bank for additional blood products including PRBCs and fresh frozen plasma (FFP).
   (c) The anesthesiologist may also prepare inotropes and pressors as boluses or infusions.
   (d) The anesthesiologist should notify the surgeon if prior to induction and intubation, they plan to better resuscitate the patient with fluids and pressors to offset the sympathectomy and hemodynamic instability that may occur with induction medications and initiation of positive pressure ventilation. The anesthesiologist may choose to administer a fluid bolus such as 20–40 cc/kg of a crystalloid solution or 10–15 cc/kg of a colloid solution.
   (e) If the anesthesiologist intends to perform these steps prior to induction, they should name a brief timeframe in which to achieve these tasks. The OB/GYN surgeon and anesthesiologist should balance these goals with the urgency of beginning surgery to control hemostasis as soon as possible.

    (f) The patient's tachycardia and hypotension will improve with this initial resuscitation.

    (g) The anesthesiologist should communicate to the OB/GYN surgeon when they are ready for induction.

    (h) The anesthesiologist should perform a rapid sequence induction and intubation.

    (i) Induction and intubation will proceed uneventfully. The airway will be secured easily. No aspiration will occur. If the previous resuscitation steps were taken prior to induction (fluid bolus, pressors, and transfusion), then the patient will sustain a small decline in blood pressure but remain within normal mean arterial pressures (MAPs).

4. Phase 3: Hemorrhage

    (a) The anesthesiologist should send labs, such as a venous blood gas (VBG) or, if they placed an arterial line, an arterial blood gas (ABG).

- Blood gas will show anemia (Hb 5.5), hypocalcemia (ionized calcium of 0.9), and metabolic acidosis (pH 7.2, $PaCO_2$ 35, PaO_2 300, and HCO_3 18).
- The anesthesiologist should recognize this and continue fluids, pressors, and blood transfusion.

    (b) The OB/GYN surgeon will have a difficult time obtaining a good view of the surgical field. There will be a large amount of blood everywhere, obstructing their view.

    (c) The team should initiate a massive transfusion protocol.

- The anesthesiologist may consider placing a central line, such as through the internal jugular vein.
- The anesthesiologist may call for a Belmont or Rapid Infuser to transfuse blood products more quickly.
- The anesthesiologist should transfuse a balanced ratio of blood products and consider cryoprecipitate.
- The anesthesiologist should send frequent ABGs and may send a CBC, coagulation panel, and thromboelastogram (TEG).

5. Phase 4: Disseminated intravascular coagulation

    (a) The patient will become increasingly tachycardic and hypotensive.

    (b) The OB/GYN surgeon will note that the blood looks very "watery."

    (c) The patient will have watery blood oozing out from their PIV and arterial line sites. The dressings over their vascular access will become loose and start to come off.

    (d) The patient will start to drop their oxygen saturation and their $ETCO_2$.

    (e) The anesthesiologist should survey their ventilator settings and circuit, increase to 100% FiO_2, hand bag ventilate to assess compliance and auscultate. They will find that there is reduced compliance on manual bagging and crackles bilaterally.

(f) The OB/GYN surgeon will identify a large tear in the cervix as the source of the rapid bleeding.

(g) The OB/GYN surgeon and anesthesiologist should discuss these findings. The team should recognize that the patient likely has disseminated intravascular coagulation (DIC). They should discuss possible etiologies, such as coagulopathy due to not maintaining a balanced transfusion of blood products such as PRBCs, FFP, platelets, and cryoprecipitate. They should also consider an AFE, given the identified cervical tear.

6. Phase 5: Right heart strain

(a) The patient will become increasingly tachycardic and begin to have brief runs of ventricular tachycardia with a pulse.

(b) The anesthesiologist should call for a crash cart with an automated external defibrillator (AED) to be brought to the room. The anesthesiologist should place pads on the patient in case of the need to deliver cardioversion.

(c) The OB/GYN surgeon will be able to repair the cervical tear quickly but will note that the patient continues to ooze watery blood. This will improve with a balanced ratio of massive transfusion.

(d) The anesthesiologist should have a strong suspicion for right heart failure due to AFE. The anesthesiologist may consider performing a TTE or TEE. If they do an echocardiogram, it will show evidence of right heart strain, including a D-shaped right ventricle, septal bowing of the interventricular septum from the right ventricle to the left ventricle, tricuspid regurgitation, dilated right ventricle, and dilated right atrium.

(e) The anesthesiologist should continue to provide inotropic support and may try to hyperventilate the patient with 100% FiO_2 to minimize pulmonary vascular resistance.

(f) The TEG will result in showing a delayed R time, K time, and alpha angle, consistent with hypo-coagulopathy.

(g) The anesthesiologist should continue a balanced transfusion.

7. Phase 6: Disposition

(a) As the team continues these supportive measures, the patient's hemodynamics will improve.

(b) Surgical hemostasis will be achieved.

(c) The OB/GYN surgeon and anesthesiologist should recap the events and current state of the resuscitation. This will include a status update on hemodynamic stability and recent labs (e.g., worsening versus improving anemia, thrombocytopenia, coagulopathy, or metabolic acidosis).

(d) The OB/GYN surgeon and anesthesiologist should discuss disposition. They may decide the patient is stable enough to be extubated. They may plan for disposition to a monitored bed with closer nursing care, such as an intensive care unit, for closer observation and continued resuscitation.

(e) The scenario will end here.

Anesthesiology Scoring Rubric

Topic: Amniotic fluid embolism		Completed	Not completed
Participants:			
Evaluators:			
Score:			
Tasks		Completed	Not completed
Phase 1: Initial survey			
Communication	Ask surgeons for additional information: Past medical history, history of present illness, current vascular access, resuscitation measures implemented so far, recent labs, blood products available, current blood loss, predicted additional blood loss, and source of bleed.		
	Discuss with the surgeons the plan to establish additional access and volume resuscitate the patient prior to induction.		
Medical management	Place the patient on full monitors.		
	Establish large-bore PIV access prior to induction.		
	Consider placing an arterial line prior to induction. May also place post-induction.		
	Administer a fluid bolus and start inotropes/ vasopressors prior to induction.		
Phase 2: Induction			
Communication	Communicate with surgeons when pre-induction resuscitation is adequate and ready for induction.		
Medical management	Perform rapid sequence induction and intubation.		
Phase 3: Hemorrhage			
Communication	Notify the surgeon that the patient remains hemodynamically unstable.		
Medical management	Escalate fluid resuscitation, transfusion, and pressors/inotropes.		
	Initiate massive transfusion protocol (MTP).		
	Transfuse blood products in a balanced ratio: PRBC, FFP, consider platelets and/or cryoprecipitate.		
	Obtain frequent ABGs to guide resuscitation.		
	Send additional labs, such as TEG, coagulation panel, CBC, and lactate.		
	Call for Belmont or rapid infuser to infuse products faster.		
Phase 4: Disseminated intravascular coagulation			
Communication	Notify the surgeon about clinical findings suggestive of DIC and coagulopathy.		
	Discuss with the surgeon possible etiologies of DIC, coagulopathy: Compromise in maternal circulation where amniotic fluid could enter; imbalanced transfusion of blood products.		

(continued)

Topic: Amniotic fluid embolism			
Medical management	Identify worsening oxygenation and ventilation. Survey ventilator and circuit, check compliance, and auscultate breath sounds. Recognize likely pulmonary edema. Recognize signs of likely DIC and coagulopathy.		
Phase 5: Right heart strain			
Communication	Notify the surgeon about the arrhythmia occurring: Ventricular tachycardia with a pulse. Notify the surgeon about evidence of right heart strain. Discuss with the surgeon the suspected diagnosis of AFE.		
Medical management	Call for a crash cart and defibrillator to be brought to the room. Place pads on the patient. Call for a TEE or TTE to be brought to the OR. Identify signs of right heart strain on echocardiogram: D-shaped right ventricle; septal bowing; tricuspid regurgitation; dilated right atrium and right ventricle. Recognize TEG showing hypo-coagulopathy. Continue balanced transfusion. Administer inotropes to support the right heart. Recognize that the DIC and right heart strain are consistent with AFE.		
Phase 6: Disposition			
Communication	Debrief with surgeons: Current hemodynamic stability, EBL, most recent labs, products given, status of resuscitation. Discuss disposition planning, including whether to remain intubated.		
Medical management	Transport to ICU for further evaluation and care.		

Septic Shock Due to Chorioamnionitis

16

Scott Lewis and Claire Sampankanpanich Soria

Target audience: Anesthesiology and Obstetrics & Gynecology (OB/GYN) residents.

16.1 Level of Training

– Anesthesiology resident
– OB/GYN resident

16.2 Learning Objectives

1. Review the signs and symptoms of chorioamnionitis.
2. Review the risk factors for chorioamnionitis.
3. Review the indications for cesarean section in patients with chorioamnionitis.
4. Discuss the perioperative management of chorioamnionitis requiring cesarean section.

16.3 Simulator Environment

1. Location: obstetric operating room in a tertiary care center.
2. Manikin setup:
    (a) Age: adult, obstetric if available.
    (b) Lines: 1 × 20 gauge peripheral intravenous (PIV) line.
    (c) Monitors: none initially; see available monitors below.

S. Lewis (✉) · C. S. Soria
University of California, San Diego, San Diego, CA, USA
e-mail: sjlewis@health.ucsd.edu; cssoria@health.ucsd.edu

3. Medications available:
    (a) Fluids: normal saline, lactated ringers.
    (b) Blood products: none.
    (c) Sedatives/hypnotics: propofol, etomidate.
    (d) Paralytics: succinylcholine, rocuronium.
    (e) Cardiac agents: epinephrine, phenylephrine, ephedrine, norepinephrine, atropine, sublingual nitroglycerin spray.
    (f) Local anesthetics: lidocaine, bupivacaine, chloroprocaine.
4. Equipment available:
    (a) Airway equipment: anesthesia ventilator (including circuit, mask, and suction), laryngoscope and cuffed endotracheal tubes (ETTs) of various sizes, stylet, oropharyngeal airway, nasopharyngeal airway, laryngeal mask airway (LMA), bougie. Video laryngoscope and fiberoptic bronchoscope are available if specifically requested by the learner.
    (b) Monitors available: pulse oximeter, blood pressure cuff, 3- or 5-lead electrocardiogram (EKG), $ETCO_2$ monitor. Additional monitors such as arterial line transducer, central venous pressure (CVP) transducer, and trans-esophageal echocardiogram (TEE) are available if specifically requested by the learner.
    (c) Line equipment available: arterial line kit and transducer, central line kit, PIV kits.
    (d) Crash cart with defibrillator available upon request.

16.4 Actors

1. Anesthesiologist(s)
2. Obstetrician(s)
3. Primary nurse and/or circulator nurse
4. Surgical scrub technician

16.5 Case Narrative

1. Background:
    (a) The obstetrician and anesthesiologist are covering the labor and delivery service overnight.
    (b) History of present illness (HPI): The patient is a 27-year-old G1P0 parturient who presents after a failed trial of labor at home due to intolerance of labor pain. She is otherwise healthy with expectant antenatal care. The patient reports regular contractions since yesterday that have become unbearably painful. Pain management thus far has been with private doulas and baths. She cannot specify the time of the rupture of membranes but believes her water broke sometime last night. She has an epidural that was placed soon after admission.

(c) Hospital course: The patient has had intermittent poor tracings including fetal tachycardia and bradycardia that recovered. The admission workup was negative, but the results of repeat labs are pending. She now has persistent fetal decelerations for which an emergent cesarean delivery is called.

(d) The care team and the patient start the scenario in the operating room.

2. Phase 1: Cesarean section starts

(a) The obstetrician should coordinate surgical procedures including but not limited to skin preparation instructions, surgical draping, available equipment, and notification of the neonatal intensive care team.

- The obstetrician should communicate significant events and status updates to the operating room including but not limited to surgical blockade testing, call for a timeout, skin incision, uterine incision, baby out, cord clamp, cord cut, uterine tone, and status of surgical hemostasis.
- The obstetrician will be able to deliver the baby swiftly and without complication.

(b) The anesthesiologist should apply the appropriate monitors and obtain initial vitals.

- Initial vital signs: HR 117 sinus rhythm, NIBP 85/45 (MAP 58), SpO_2 100% on room air.

(c) The anesthesiologist should assess the patient's epidural, which will reveal adequate bilateral labor analgesia.

- The anesthesiologist should immediately administer anesthetic to convert the labor epidural to adequate surgical blockade.
- The anesthesiologist should administer vasoactive medications to counteract the expected sympathectomy. The required dose will be higher than the average or expected.

(d) The patient will have minimal response to fluid boluses and vasoactive medications administered by the anesthesiologist.

- Inadequate resuscitation with fluids and vasoactive medications will precipitate rapid decompensation to phase 2 as below.
- With appropriate management, the patient's vitals will remain sinus tachycardia with MAPs 55–65.

(e) The anesthesiologist should communicate with the obstetrician that the patient is requiring more than the average amount of vasoactive medications and fluid administration to maintain blood pressure. They should inquire about surgical blood loss and/or complications.

- The obstetrician should acknowledge the anesthesiologist's communication of concerns about vasoactive support and advise of any surgical concerns that may be contributing.
- The anesthesiologist should consider and/or place an arterial line after discussion with the obstetrician.

3. Phase 2: Decompensation to septic shock

(a) The patient's clinical status will deteriorate. She will report lightheadedness, nausea, and dizziness. She will request an emesis bag and vomit. She will report feeling very warm.

(b) The anesthesiologist should reassess the vitals.
- New vitals: HR 130 sinus rhythm, NIBP 70/40 (MAP 50), SpO_2 92% on room air.
- The anesthesiologist should apply a skin temperature probe (e.g., axilla).
  - Temperature is 38.3 °C.

(c) The anesthesiologist should communicate the patient's clinical status change to the obstetrician including but not limited to vitals, current vasoactive support, and symptoms.

(d) The anesthesiologist should continue to escalate care including but not limited to: inserting additional PIV, inserting an arterial line, providing supplemental oxygen, and/or starting vasoactive or inotropic support.
- The patient will remain minimally responsive to ephedrine bolus and phenylephrine bolus/infusion.
- The patient will be appropriately responsive to norepinephrine bolus/infusion and vasopressin bolus/infusion.

(e) The anesthesiologist should evaluate for signs and symptoms of high spinal blockade and local anesthetic systemic toxicity (LAST). The patient's exam will be inconsistent with these pathologies.

(f) The patient decompensates further and becomes unresponsive.
- New vitals: HR 140 sinus rhythm, NIBP 68/30 (MAP 43), SpO_2 90% on room air (94% if the anesthesiologist is administering supplemental O_2).
- The anesthesiologist should determine that the patient requires intubation, inform the surgical team, and perform an rapid sequence induction (RSI) intubation.
- The anesthesiologist should call for help at this time if an assisting anesthesiologist is available. Alternatively, calling a code pink to rapidly obtain additional resources should be considered.

(g) The obstetrician and anesthesiologist should discuss current concerns and collaborate on a differential diagnosis given the change in clinical status.
- The obstetrician and/or anesthesiologist should inquire as to the results of the repeat laboratory evaluation, which will now be available.
  - Results: leukocytosis >15,000 × 10^6 cells/L, otherwise within normal limits, no growth on admission cultures.
- The anesthesiologist should obtain a core temperature (esophageal or nasopharyngeal).
  - Temperature is now 39 °C.
- The obstetrician should request a quantitative blood loss analysis.
- The obstetrician should request that the anesthesiologist evaluate the urine.
- The obstetrician should ask another member of the team to perform a vaginal exam to assess for bleeding.
- The patient will have a surgical field with hemostasis, normal range surgical blood loss, low volume vaginal bleeding within expected ranges, and normal volume urine output without gross evidence of blood.

(h) The obstetrician and anesthesiologist should discuss a leading diagnosis, immediate next steps, and an overall treatment plan including disposition.

- A leading diagnosis of chorioamnionitis in the setting of prolonged labor prior to admission should be reached.
- Appropriate antibiotics should be ordered and administered without delay.
  - Blood cultures should be obtained first unless it would delay antibiotic administration.
- During the disposition discussion, the anesthesiologist should include concerns about extubation given large volume resuscitation and unstable hemodynamics. A recommendation of remaining intubated and ICU level of care should be made to the obstetrician.

(i) The simulation may end here or proceed to the next phase at the discretion of the moderator(s).

4. Phase 3: Advanced cardiac life support (ACLS)/code
   (a) This phase should be incorporated unanimously for higher level learners or in response to grossly inadequate care in phase 2 at the discretion of the moderator(s).
   (b) The patient will further decompensate, become profoundly hypotensive despite intervention, and/or enter an unstable cardiac rhythm requiring ACLS.
   (c) The obstetrician and/or anesthesiologist should begin ACLS and call a code.
      - The code should be repeated if an earlier code pink was called as resources and staff would leave after no longer being needed.
      - The cardiac rhythm and progression of ACLS are at the discretion of the moderator(s).
   (d) The anesthesiologist should consider escalation of care including, but not limited to arterial line (if not already present), central line, escalation of choice, or dose of pressors and/or inotropes.
   (e) The anesthesiologist should consider the insertion of a TEE (trans-thoracic echocardiogram (TTE) unavailable given compressions). Images will be available and show an underfilled hyperdynamic heart.
   (f) If a return of spontaneous circulation (ROSC) is obtained, the anesthesiologist and obstetrician should revisit disposition and agree upon the ICU level of care.
   (g) The simulation ends here for all learners.

Anesthesiology Scoring Rubric

Topic: Septic shock due to chorioamnionitis			
Participants:			
Evaluators:			
Score:			
Tasks		Completed	Not completed
Phase 1: Cesarean section starts			
Communication	Advise obstetrician of patient's fluid bolus and vasoactive meds resistant hypotension.		
	Ask about surgical blood loss vs. complications.		
Medical management	Apply monitors (at least EKG, pulse oximeter, NIBP cuff).		
	Obtain baseline vitals (cycle NIBP cuff).		
	Assess the patient's labor epidural.		
	Convert labor epidural to surgical block without delay.		
	Administer vasoactive support for sympathectomy.		
	Administer a fluid bolus in response to hypotension.		
	Escalate vasoactive support of hypotension (dose or medication change).		
Phase 2: Decompensation to septic shock			
Communication	Advise obstetrician of clinical status change.		
	Advise obstetrician of deteriorating vitals and new fever.		
	Advise obstetrician that patient is unresponsive and of the decision to intubate.		
	Request surgical field status update (blood loss, tone, complications).		
	Discuss concerns and differential diagnosis with an obstetrician (septic shock must be included).		
	Discuss disposition (ICU, remain intubated).		
Medical management	Reassess vitals in response to clinical status change (nausea/vomiting, dizziness).		
	Evaluate for high spinal blockade.		
	Evaluate for local anesthetic systemic toxicity (LAST).		
	Apply skin temperature probe.		
	Insert additional PIV.		
	Insert arterial line.		
	Escalate vasoactive support (must be medication change) or start the inotropic agent.		
	Administer 30 mL/kg fluid bolus.		
	Intubate patients without delay after they become unresponsive.		
	Call for help (may be done in phase 1).		
	Requests results of repeat labs.		
	Obtains core temperature.		

(continued)

Topic: Septic shock due to chorioamnionitis		
Phase 3: ACLS/code		
Communication	Advise the entire care team patient is increasingly unstable.	
	Report loss of pulses, call a code pink.	
	Run the code as the team leader.	
	Coordinate resources including delegation of tasks.	
	Confirm disposition to ICU after ROSC (if obtained).	
Medical management	Start ACLS.	
	Follow the appropriate algorithmic pathway for the clinical scenario (per moderator's choice, such as pulseless electrical activity and ventricular tachycardia).	
	Insert arterial line (if not done earlier).	
	Insert central line.	
	Start inotropic support as appropriate.	
	Insert and evaluate TEE (TTE unavailable given compressions).	

Index

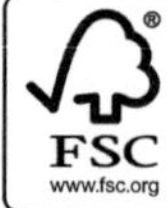

MIX
Papier aus verantwortungsvollen Quellen
Paper from responsible sources
FSC® C105338

If you have any concerns about our products,
you can contact us on
ProductSafety@springernature.com

In case Publisher is established outside the EU,
the EU authorized representative is:
Springer Nature Customer Service Center GmbH
Europaplatz 3, 69115 Heidelberg, Germany

Printed by Libri Plureos GmbH
in Hamburg, Germany